Complete College Cookbook

COMPLETE
COLLEGE
COOKBOOK

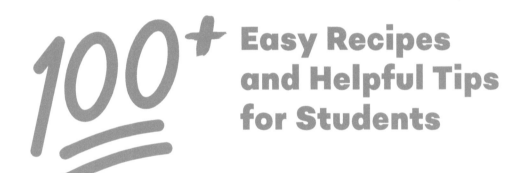

100+ Easy Recipes and Helpful Tips for Students

Julee Morrison

ROCKRIDGE
PRESS

For general information on our other products and services or to obtain technical support, please contact our Customer Care Department within the United States at (866) 744-2665, or outside the United States at (510) 253-0500.

Rockridge Press publishes its books in a variety of electronic and print formats. Some content that appears in print may not be available in electronic books, and vice versa.

TRADEMARKS: Rockridge Press and the Rockridge Press logo are trademarks or registered trademarks of Callisto Media Inc. and/or its affiliates, in the United States and other countries, and may not be used without written permission. All other trademarks are the property of their respective owners. Rockridge Press is not associated with any product or vendor mentioned in this book.

Interior and Cover Designer: Erik Jacobsen
Art Producer: Hannah Dickerson
Editor: Rebecca Markley
Production Editor: Jenna Dutton
Production Manager: Riley Hoffman

Photography © 2021 Emulsion Studio, cover and p. VIII; © Emulsion Studio, back cover (all except second from left) and pp. 28, 56, 120, 140; © Darren Muir, back cover (second from left) and p. 156; © Heidi's Bridge, pp. X, 98; © Paul Sirisalee, pp. 12, 72; © Marija Vidal, p. 40. Icons and patterns used throughout under license from iStock.com. Author photo courtesy of MacKenzie Morrison.

ISBN: Print 978-1-63807-311-6
        eBook 978-1-63807-137-2
R0

This book is dedicated to Kyra and Jake—
our first college graduates. xoxo

Contents

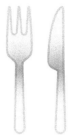

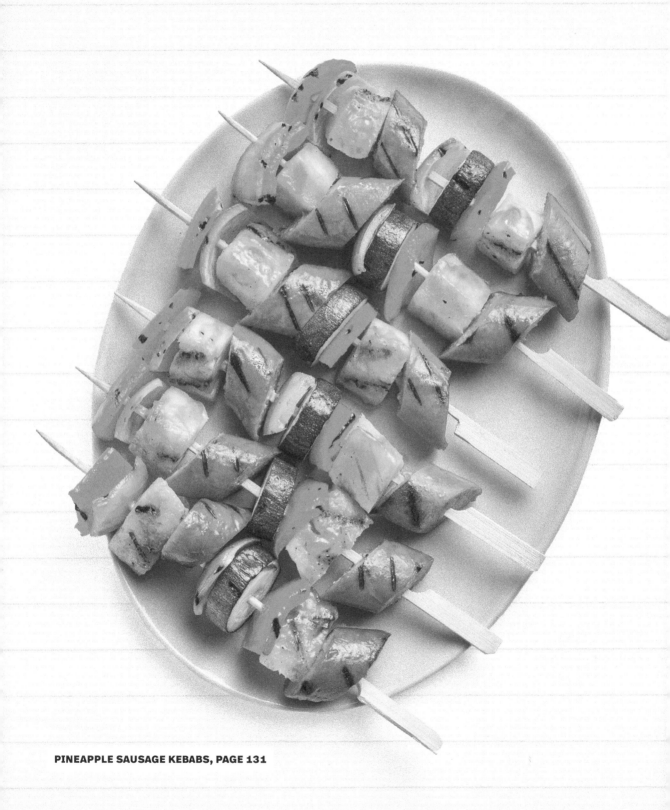

PINEAPPLE SAUSAGE KEBABS, PAGE 131

Introduction

Welcome to *Complete College Cookbook*. I look forward to spending time "together" preparing delicious meals and snacks to help power you through college study sessions, introduce you to entertaining, and encourage you in a potential new hobby: cooking.

I am a casual chef. I am also an adventurous one. I like easy, laid-back recipes, but I also like trying new recipes with different tastes and techniques, so I might make a recipe or two each month that challenges my cooking style. I have two college graduates of my own and another child who is in her sophomore year. As a result, I have witnessed the food options available on many college campuses and have also seen firsthand the constraints of cooking as a student: Time management is crucial. You have a limited budget. You're operating within a small work space, sometimes just a desk.

This book takes into account the fact that you need recipes that are quick and easy so that you can make it to class. It recognizes that grocery shopping isn't where you want to spend your time. The recipes here cater to intense study sessions and offer nutritious, brain-fueling snacks and dinners for one. But, of course, what is college without socializing? This cookbook includes two chapters, Meals with Friends (page 99) and Tailgating and Party Food (page 121), specifically so you can cook for your friends.

Whether you have a couple of recipes in your rotation or have never cooked before in your life, this cookbook will help you prepare healthy and delicious meals without taking up too much time, money, equipment, or space. My hope in writing this book is that it will inspire you to start cooking more, leading you to an appreciation of cooking and many fulfilling meals in your future.

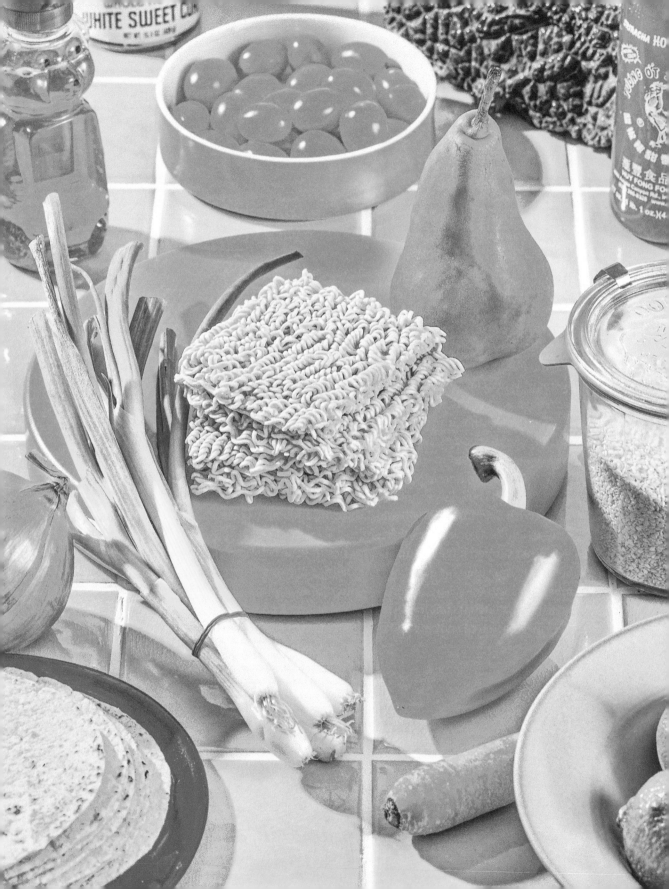

1

Setting Up Your College Kitchen

Do not let limited space intimidate you. This chapter presents an approach to cooking in your dorm room or apartment with limited ingredients and even more limited equipment. Many of the recipes in this book are no-bake or microwave only. As long as you can find a small amount of space for canned goods and spices, deli meats, and mason jars, you'll be good to go.

Cooking for All the Right Reasons

Sure, cold cereal will get you through a couple hours, and takeout is fun once or twice a week, but having something warm and freshly cooked will increase your focus, fuel you throughout your day, and have your body working at its optimal capacity. Cooking puts you in control of what goes into your body and when: It is healthier than ordering fast food and, even if you have a meal plan, the dining hall may be closed when you have the time to eat. Cooking is cost effective and will help you avoid the extra pounds that fast food, junk food, and a lot of dining hall food can quickly add to your body. If you know how to cook, even basic recipes, you will not go hungry. And college is a great time to start, even with (or especially with) the limited space, time, and access to equipment and groceries.

You are going to have cooking fails, and that's okay. It's part of the process. Learn from them and move on. The more you cook, the more your cooking will evolve. Simple techniques will help you build the foundation for more complicated techniques. This book will teach you the basics of cooking in a small space, on which you can expand as you move into your own apartment and begin cooking for more than just yourself.

Food is universal; it's the flavors that change. As you develop your skills, you'll be excited to share them with others. When I was in college, I had a group of friends who were all learning to cook. We would have one weekend a month with a theme, like Mexican food, and each person would bring their favorite dish for that theme. It was a night of fun, but we also taught each other about spices, techniques, and garnish. Plus, cooking and eating together cements friendships.

FIVE DISHES EVERY COLLEGE STUDENT SHOULD COOK

This book covers a range of foods to satisfy your many moods and cravings. Midnight snacks? Check. Tailgating munchies? Check. Vegan breakfasts? Check. But here are five recipes worth highlighting because they are universally popular, and you'll be able to master them in no time flat.

Overnight Oats (remix tip, page 38); With minimal preparation the night before, you will wake up to this delicious and filling breakfast. It is ready to grab and go on those mornings you need to dash out the door.

Chicken Parmesan (page 83): Recreate a taste of home. Breaded chicken breasts smothered in cheese offer a protein power kick. Add an easy marinara and pasta, and you have a delicious, satisfying meal.

Charcuterie Board (page 49): These boards offer so many options for snacking. Whether you're craving sweet or savory, a charcuterie board has you covered. It also contains the protein, variety, and texture you need to get through that study session and keep you and your friends focused.

Cobb Salad (page 60): Your favorite salad ready to go. Fill a mason jar with all the layers of a Cobb salad—bacon, chicken, egg, tomatoes, avocado, corn, and black beans—add some dressing, and give it a shake.

Grilled Burgers (page 123): Delicious burgers on the grill. Perfect for game days and gatherings with friends. Set up a condiment station and get your grub on.

College Kitchen Essentials

You do not need the perfect kitchen to create the perfect meal. College cooking is at its best in a small space and using a small number of simple tools and appliances to their full potential. You'll become resourceful and flexible as a chef. Here, you'll discover the kitchen essentials that will help you make the most of your small space and limited time to create food that is big on taste.

Some appliances might require a small outlay of cash; however, they are investments that will pay for themselves quickly as you learn to cook. They also will last beyond your college years. Check thrift stores and yard sales, or just ask around, and you may find these essentials at deeply discounted prices or free. You do not have to own everything suggested at once. Start with a few recipes, and as your comfort level increases, add a new item and a new recipe into your rotation. Check around the dorm as well. Some of these tools may be available to borrow or share.

Tools

Can Opener: For opening canned goods. Look for one with a comfortable grip.

Meat Thermometer: A digital meat thermometer takes the guesswork out of cooking meat. For the perfect medium-rare steak, you want 145°F, for instance. For tender, juicy chicken, safe from salmonella, cook to 165°F.

Small (6-inch) Skillet: A small skillet is useful for making omelets, sandwiches, sauces, and smaller dishes.

Large (10-inch) Skillet: A large skillet is a necessity for browning meats and other ingredients that need space to cook properly.

3-Quart Saucepan with Lid: A medium saucepan is great for making sauces, cooking vegetables, and boiling eggs.

8-Quart Saucepan with Lid: This kitchen essential is perfect for soups, pasta, puddings, and more.

Paring Knife: Use a paring knife for peeling vegetables and fruit, deseeding fruit, deveining shrimp, cutting vegetables, and precision work.

Chef's Knife: This multipurpose knife will cut meat, chop vegetables, and perform a variety of kitchen tasks.

Cutting Boards: Ideally, you want one cutting board for vegetables and another for meats. Plastic is great for meats, while wood works well for fruits and vegetables. Look for boards that are easy to clean and sanitize.

Resealable Containers: These containers are helpful for eating on the go, reheating leftovers, and storing foods. Look for a set that comes with a variety of sizes.

Measuring Cups: Look for a set of measuring cups that nest neatly together to maximize space. You'll want a set of at least four, from ¼ cup to 1 cup. For measuring liquids, you will need a cup with graduated measurement lines. A sturdy glass measuring cup can even be used in the microwave.

Measuring Spoons: Ideally, your measuring spoons should nest together, too. Look for a set of six that includes sizes from ⅛ teaspoon to 1 tablespoon.

Mixing Bowls: Your mixing bowls should also nest together to save space. A set of three bowls—small, medium, and large—is great for mixing ingredients, tossing salads, marinating meat, serving, and more.

Rimmed Baking Sheet: Use a baking sheet for baking cookies or roasting meats and vegetables. The rimmed edges will keep liquids from dripping to the bottom of the oven.

8-by-8-Inch Baking Pan: This square baking pan is the perfect size for roasting smaller portions of meat and vegetables, as well as baking cakes and brownies.

Silicone Spatula: A silicone spatula can be used to stir, scrape the sides of a bowl while mixing, spread ingredients, or lift food.

Microwave-Safe Dishes: A microwave-safe dish is one that, when you add water and heat in the microwave for one minute, is still cool to the touch.

Oven Mitts: With oven mitts, you can handle a hot pan in a safe manner.

Equipment

Microwave: This must-have appliance can be used for both cooking and reheating foods. This cookbook utilizes the microwave for many recipes.

Toaster Oven: This multipurpose kitchen workhorse can make toast, heat leftovers, and even cook full dishes.

Hot Plate or Single Burner: A hot plate takes up little space yet allows you to cook almost anything you would on a traditional stove top.

Electric Pressure Cooker: This multipurpose appliance can serve as a pressure cooker, slow cooker, rice cooker, yogurt maker, and more.

Blender: This handy appliance takes up little space. It requires minimal knowledge to operate and can help in preparing smoothies, pancake mix, protein shakes, gravy, fruit purees, and more.

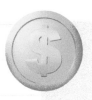

HOW TO SAVE MONEY
WHILE SHOPPING

Being on a tight budget doesn't mean you won't be able to equip your college kitchen. Stretch your budget while learning to cook.

→ Familiarize yourself with weekly store circulars that feature sale items. Many stores also offer a student discount.

→ Sign up for store reward programs. You can get customer discounts, earn points toward gas, and get valuable coupons by joining.

→ Pay attention to school bulletin boards; someone may be offering heavily discounted appliances or kitchen tools.

→ Browse yard sales and estate sales, both online and in person, for the items on your list.

→ Store brands offer quality products. Save money by choosing the store brand over the name brand.

→ Shop online sales for savings. Visit brand social media pages and websites to see if they have coupons to apply toward purchases.

→ Share what you are looking for with family and friends, and ask them to keep you in mind if they find a deal.

→ Wait for holiday sales like Black Friday, Cyber Monday, Amazon Prime Day, Small Business Day, and after-holiday discounts for savings.

Mini Fridge: This is a great small appliance in your dorm room for chilling fresh produce, eggs, condiments, milk, and leftovers. You can even use the top of it as a meal prep area to maximize space.

Ingredient Essentials

Many inexpensive and easily accessible ingredients that will help you become a great college cook are featured in the recipes in this cookbook. This chapter will help you get your ingredient essentials in order, including the right spices, must-have pantry items, and making the most of your mini fridge.

Pantry

Rice and Pasta: These are great staples to have because they go with almost everything. These are inexpensive but filling options for a main or side dish.

Canned Beans: Beans are a versatile staple and an excellent plant-based protein. Consider black beans, pintos, refried beans, kidney beans, and garbanzo beans (also known as chickpeas).

Spices: You can usually buy a spice rack with spices already included. The spices most used in this book include black pepper, garlic powder, thyme, cinnamon, oregano, rosemary, cayenne pepper, cumin, and paprika.

Spice Blends: Spice blends offer a combination of spices in one container, which can save money and time. If you lean toward Italian dishes, look for Italian or Mediterranean seasoning blends.

Salt: There are so many types of salt, and they do bring different things to the table (literally), but for these recipes you can use table salt, which is the most affordable option.

Oil: Oil is a necessity for dressings and keeping your food from sticking to the pan. Many recipes in this book use extra-virgin olive oil, which is full of healthy fats.

Tomato Sauce: This versatile staple makes a great marinara sauce.

Quick Oats: Quick-cooking oats are for more than just oatmeal—use them in cookies, meatloaf, and more.

Canned Meats: Tuna, chicken, and ham are great options for quick sandwich fillings or salad toppers, and you can add them to soups, rice, and more.

All-Purpose Flour: Plain white flour is the starter for many recipes. It can be used to make batters, coat meats for pan-frying, and thicken sauces and gravies.

Nut and Seed Butters: Peanut, almond, cashew, and sunflower butters are delicious and packed with protein.

Refrigerator

Eggs: Eggs are versatile and an excellent source of protein. Fry them, boil them, poach them, scramble them, or use them as a binding agent.

Dairy, Nut, or Soy Milk: Milk is used to soften foods, add flavor, and moisten dry ingredients.

Butter: Smeared on bread or used in a recipe, butter adds volume, flavor, and texture, and prevents sticking.

Leafy Greens: These affordable vegetables are packed with vitamins and nutrients, and can be eaten raw or cooked.

Cheese: Cheese is a great snack on its own or can be grated, shredded, sliced, or diced for all kinds of recipes. It is a good source of calcium and protein.

Condiments: Soy sauce, mayonnaise, mustard, ketchup, vinegar, hot sauce, salad dressings, barbecue sauce, and Worcestershire sauce are all condiments that add a pop of flavor to any dish. See chapter 10, Staples (page 157), to find out how to make some of these condiments yourself.

Deli Meats: Salami, pepperoni, sliced turkey, sliced ham, and bologna can be used in sandwiches, in wraps, on charcuterie boards, and added to casseroles and soups.

Yogurt: Yogurt is a great snack or quick breakfast, and a good source of calcium.

Jam/Jelly: Sure, jam is great on sandwiches, but it can also be a glaze for meats, a topping for baked goods, and more.

BRAIN FOOD

Not all foods are created equal. Some are better at fueling your body and brain for those long lectures, all-night study sessions, and lengthy term papers. Look for foods that are high in protein, complex carbohydrates, omega-3s, antioxidants, and monounsaturated fats. Try these recipes for their blend of brain power and deliciousness.

Wild Rice and Baked Salmon (page 85): This dish offers protein and omega-3s. It is not only delicious but loaded with the nutrients your brain needs for mental clarity and concentration.

Banana-Berry Smoothie Bowl (page 35): This yummy combination of fruits and nuts offers complex carbohydrates, omega-3s, antioxidants, and plant protein for better brain function and more energy.

Easy Chicken Salad (page 58): Nuts provide energy, and chicken adds protein. Both are excellent choices to power the brain with focus and improve memory. Use a whole-wheat wrap to release energy slowly and avoid the crash.

Guacamole (page 46): Mix up some guacamole and enjoy the benefits of its healthy monounsaturated fats, which enhance problem-solving and memory.

Bean-y Burrito Bowl (page 71): This recipe is an excellent source of protein. Add avocado and you have a bowl that is ready to take on a serious study session. It keeps your brain performing and your stomach full.

Cottage Cheese and Spinach Scrambled Eggs (page 33): Your brain will reap the benefits of choline, vitamin K, protein, and healthy fats, which boost memory and improve the brain's ability to focus and problem solve.

Making the Most of Your Mini Fridge

You have limited space in your mini fridge, so it's important to maximize it and keep an eye on what you already have and need to use up.

Eliminate Excess Packaging: Consider repackaging items in smaller containers—but don't forget to save the directions. Cut the directions from the box and stick them to your mini fridge with a magnet.

Store Fruits and Vegetables: Storage makes a difference for fruits and vegetables. In a pantry, apples last three weeks, whereas they can last four to six weeks in a refrigerator. Keep in mind that storing fruits and vegetables together makes them ripen faster and reduces their lifespan. This is due to ethylene, a gas that most fruits produce.

Pay Attention to Color and Texture: Green vegetables turning yellow, potatoes turning green, meat turning dark brown, and poultry turning gray are all signs that the food is no longer good to eat. Meats, poultry, and fish should be moist, not sticky or slimy.

Pay Attention to Packaging: If food packaging bulges, is dented, or has an "off" odor or appearance, it is best to discard rather than risk getting sick.

Understand Those "xxx-By" Dates: Use-By is the date by which the product should be eaten. Best-By is a suggestion for consuming the product and assuring quality. The expiration date is the date beyond which you should not use the product.

Time to Start Cooking

Throughout this book, you will learn about flavors, discover easy recipes to feed yourself, and find ways to share your cooking skills with friends. A little advance planning will maximize your time and help you stick to a budget without sacrificing variety and flavor. Even if you plan to cook only two or three times a week, if you do it consistently, you will notice steady progress in your skills.

In the next chapter, I will share techniques to help you approach cooking as a college student. The most important tool is your open mind; if you are open to trying new things, you'll find a world of food options to bring comfort on a rainy day, power you through a difficult study session, or bond with your friends.

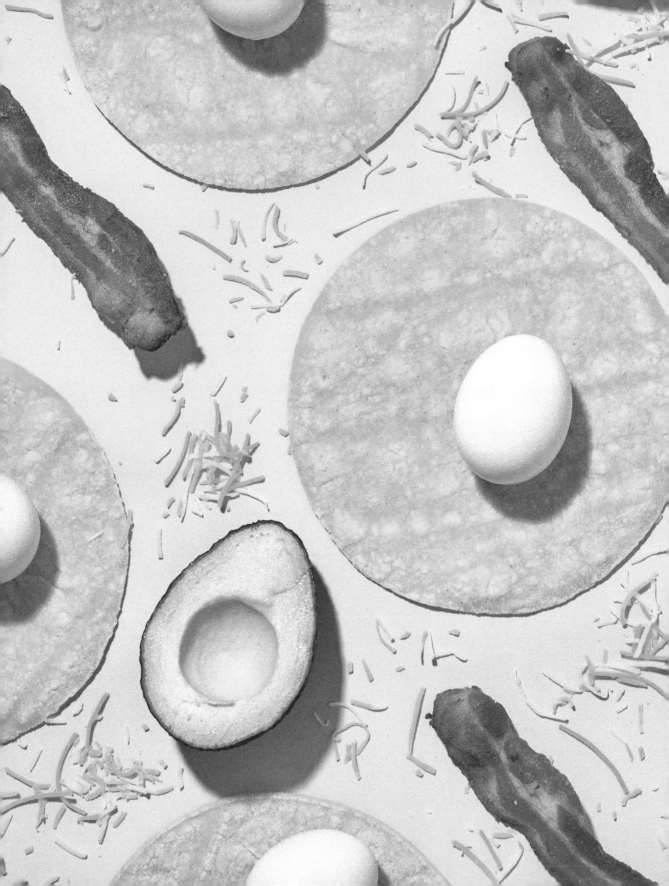

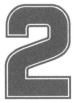

A Crash Course in College Cooking

Before we get started on the recipes, this chapter will provide some quick information on cooking techniques, the use of various kitchen appliances, and successfully cooking a recipe in a dorm room or small kitchen.

The Seven Skills You Need to Cook in College

The great thing about cooking is that you learn as you go. You aren't going to start out as a culinary expert, but this book will help you learn the basic skills that will come in handy.

Holding a Knife Properly: Hold the knife like you are shaking hands with it. Use your dominant hand and curl your fingers around the handle of the knife. Your thumb should be over the knife handle, and your grip should be underneath. It is important to grip the handle so you have the greatest control over the knife. Keep your hand behind the bolster (where the handle meets the blade) when handling the knife. Only cut on a flat surface.

Slicing: When you are slicing, you cut across the grain into thin, uniform pieces. Hold the knife and pull backward slowly at an even angle; there should be no downward movement. The entire length of the blade should slice through the food.

Chopping/Dicing: Use downward motions with a knife to cut food into pieces. Chopping typically means larger pieces, whereas dicing means to chop into smaller pieces. A chef's knife works best for both.

Measuring: Measuring is one major key to your cooking success. For dry ingredients, use cups or spoons leveled off with a kitchen knife. Liquids are measured in a cup marked with graduated lines of measurement, placed on a level surface, and filled to the desired line. If you're using the same cup for dry and wet ingredients, measure dry ingredients first, then oils, then liquids.

Mixing: When you take the time to mix dry ingredients separately from wet ingredients, and then combine wet and dry ingredients together, your recipe will have a more consistent texture and flavor.

Stirring: On a stove top, you stir (blend ingredients using a circular motion) to keep ingredients moving for even cooking. In a bowl, you stir to create a uniform mixture. **Stir continuously** means you stir with no breaks, typically to thicken a liquid or prevent it from scorching. **Stir frequently** is usually for solids being added to a liquid—like flour to broth to make a gravy by reduction; you stir here and there with breaks in between. **Stir occasionally** is stirring just enough to keep the heat even and prevent the food from burning.

Tossing: Use a light lift-and-drop method. You lift up the food and gently flip it over as you drop it gently back into the bowl or pan.

TALK LIKE A CHEF

I like to think of the kitchen as its own territory with its own language. Here are 15 common terms you will come across in these recipes and whenever you are cooking.

Beat: To incorporate air and make a mixture smooth by mixing rapidly by hand or with an electric mixer

Blend: To mix two or more ingredients together

Chill: To put food in the refrigerator until completely cold

Cool: To allow hot or warm food to drop to room temperature

Drizzle: To pour a liquid back and forth over food in a fine stream

Fold: To combine foods, usually light ingredients into heavier ingredients, using a spatula in an over-and-under motion

Grease: To coat the interior of a pan with a fat, like butter or oil, to prevent food from sticking during the cooking process

Marinate: To soak food (usually meat) in a flavored liquid

Preheat: To heat the oven to a specified temperature before putting the food in to cook

Puree: To blend food with a blender until completely smooth

Sauté: To quickly cook chopped foods until cooked through and lightly browned to preserve flavor and texture

Sear: To cook food at a high temperature until a brown crust forms

Season: To add salt, pepper, or spices to a food

Simmer: To cook in liquid just below the boiling point; bubbles will break at the surface more slowly than at a full boil

Whisk: To beat ingredients like eggs, salad dressing, or heavy cream with a fork or whisk to mix, blend, or incorporate air

Cooking with the Almighty Microwave

Because dorm rooms are small, and because there are rules, sometimes the only appliance allowed is a microwave. For that reason, many of the recipes in this book utilize the microwave.

You can use the microwave not only for reheating food but for cooking, steaming, crisping, melting, and more. Many conventional cooking techniques are the same in a microwave. For greater success, pay attention to how food is arranged and processed: When cooking meats, the thickest part of the meat should be on the outside of the dish. More delicate foods like asparagus tips should be pointed toward the inside of the dish. When cooking meat or baked potatoes, flip the food during cooking to ensure it cooks evenly. If you are cooking multiple items, they should be placed in a circular arrangement with a space between them. Rearrange the items, rotating those on the outside to the center of the dish, and vice versa, partway through cooking to promote even cooking.

Always allow foods to stand after they finish in the microwave. This "rest time" completes the cooking and allows heat to disperse evenly. The rest time will depend on the surface area and the density of the food item.

Some of my favorite microwave recipes include Microwave Oatmeal (page 38), Microwave Nachos Three Ways (page 44), Microwave Macaroni and Cheese (page 82), Microwave Peach Chicken (page 105), and Apple Spice Mug Cake (page 143).

Rice and Pasta in the Microwave

If you know how to make these two staples in the microwave, you can make meals for weeks in your dorm room.

How to Make Rice in the Microwave

Prep time: 2 minutes **Cook time:** 15 minutes, plus 5 minutes to rest
Total time: 22 minutes

Makes 3 cups
1 cup short-grain rice
2 cups water
½ teaspoon salt
1 teaspoon butter

1. In a 2-quart microwave-safe dish, combine the rice, water, salt, and butter, and cover.

2. Microwave on high for 15 minutes.

3. Let the rice rest for 5 minutes, then remove it from the microwave. Lift the cover and fluff with fork.

How to Make Pasta in the Microwave

Prep time: 2 minutes **Cook time:** 18 minutes **Total time:** 20 minutes

4 cups water
8 ounces pasta

1. In a 3-quart microwave-safe dish, pour in the water and cover.

2. Microwave on high for 8 minutes to bring the water to a slow boil.

3. Add the pasta to the dish of boiling water, stir to break up the noodles, and cover.

4. Microwave on high for 10 minutes, or until tender, stirring once.

5. Drain the noodles.

What to Avoid in the Microwave

Here are some basic microwave don'ts: Never put metal in the microwave, including metal pans or dishes with metallic trim, handles, or screws; paper-covered metal twist-ties; or foil-lined packages. Do not put melamine dinnerware in the microwave.

As for plastics, if they are dishwasher safe, they should be okay in the microwave for shorter cooking times. Never use plastic for tomato-based foods or those with a high fat or sugar content. Tomatoes will stain plastic containers because of a molecule in the tomato called lycopene. It dissolves into the plastic and stains it. High-fat and high-sugar content foods heat more quickly and to higher temperatures than other foods and can quickly melt plastic.

How to Clean the Microwave

Clean the microwave after each use. You can use a damp paper towel to wipe down the inside. For messier microwaves, pour 1 cup of water into a microwave-safe bowl and add 1 drop dish soap. Place in the microwave and heat uncovered for 5 minutes. Let sit in the microwave for 3 minutes, then remove the dish and wipe the inside of the microwave with a damp cloth.

All About Toaster Ovens

While toaster ovens are not allowed in many dorm rooms, the common area may have one, or you may be able to bring your own to use in the common area. You can, of course, use a toaster oven to toast breads, reheat foods, and crisp them up, but there are numerous other great uses for a toaster oven as well.

A toaster oven is great for recipes like Mushroom Cheesesteaks (page 70), Buffalo Toaster Oven Chicken Sliders (page 80), and Chicken Parmesan (page 83). It is also the perfect vehicle for Avocado Toast (page 32) and the many varieties of avocado toast, as well as Toaster Oven Caramelized Bacon (page 51). But don't let me stop you there. You can make baked potatoes for a potato bar and potato slices to crisp and serve with Parmesan cheese. You can put tablespoons of macaroni and cheese on aluminum foil, add some bread crumbs and butter, and create delectable mac and cheese balls. You can even make roasted chicken wings. The toaster oven allows you to make small batches. Basically, you can use a toaster oven for anything you would use a broiler for when cooking.

SEVEN MIRACULOUS MICROWAVE HACKS

Sure, the microwave gets a lot of use nuking frozen burritos, but it has other uses that may not be so obvious. Some of them are cooking-related, while others are simply "life hacks."

Peel Garlic Without the Mess: After microwaving a whole head of garlic for 30 seconds, the cloves will simply pop out without any of the skin sticking to your knife or fingers.

Melt Butter: Put butter in a small bowl and cook on high in 20-second intervals, until melted.

Soften Brown Sugar: Put an apple slice in a bag of hardened brown sugar and microwave on high for 5 seconds.

Warm Towels: This is a great face refresher during long study sessions. Put dampened washcloths in a microwavable dish and microwave on high for 1 to 3 minutes, just until warm.

Roast Nuts: Put nuts in a single layer on a plate and microwave them for 1 minute. Repeat until the nuts are roasted to your liking.

Peel Fruits and Vegetables: Peaches and tomatoes work best for this hack, which makes peeling them easier. Cut the fruit in half, put it on a plate, and microwave it in 10-second intervals until the skin wrinkles. Peel the microwaved fruit with a fork.

A Blender for All Seasons

Blenders are great because they reduce prep time in the kitchen and create delicious smoothies, soups, salsa, and drinks. When using a blender, begin by placing the container firmly on the small stud at the base center and locking it into place. Put ingredients in the container, cover, and select your speed or the function for what you are making. To clean the blender, fill the container halfway with hot water, add a few drops of dish soap, and cover. Blend for 30 seconds on medium speed. Rinse and dry the container. Keep in mind that you should never use boiling liquids (or any liquid above 180°F) in the blender with the lid closed. Hot liquid creates steam, which creates pressure, and pressure can cause an explosion.

In this book, I have created many smoothie recipes, like the Green Power Smoothie Bowl (page 36), and numerous other blended recipes, like 20-Second Homemade Mayonnaise (page 158) and Cheese Ball (page 47). But one of my favorite uses for the blender is chocolate sauce. It is perfect as an ice cream topping, stirred into milk for hot cocoa, added to coffee for a body-warming mocha, or as a dip for cookies.

Less-Than-Two-Minute Blender Chocolate Sauce

Prep time: 1 minute 30 seconds

6 ounces semisweet chocolate chips

⅓ cup hot tap water (not over 180°F)

1. Put the chocolate chips in the blender.

2. Pour in the hot tap water and cover.

3. Blend for 20 seconds on high speed and consume to your heart's content.

Getting the Most Out of Pots and Pans

"Pans" typically refer to flat, shallow cookware, such as frying pans and baking sheets. Frying pans are used to cook eggs, bacon, pancakes, steaks, and similar items. Baking sheets are perfect for cookies and other baked items, or dishes like nachos. "Pots" (also called "saucepans") are typically deeper and are used to cook sauces and soups, and to boil pasta.

Here are some general tips for working with pots and pans. It is best to let your pan heat up slowly for one to two minutes before you begin cooking. This will help you cook more evenly and reduce cooking time. Always let your pots and pans cool down naturally; avoid putting a hot pan in water because it can warp. If you are boiling pasta or soup, rest a wooden spoon across the pan. This will prevent it from boiling over. Wooden spoons and spatulas are the best tools to stir food in pots and pans (especially nonstick pans) because they won't scratch the surfaces. Nonstick cooking spray is a great tool in the kitchen. You can spray it lightly in your pots and pans before cooking to prevent sticking.

In this book, some of the recipes you'll discover that use pans include Easy French Toast (page 31), Cottage Cheese and Spinach Scrambled Eggs (page 33), Cheese Quesadilla (page 50), and Herb-Crusted Salmon (page 110). Recipes that use pots include Chicken Noodle Soup (page 107), and Tailgate Three-Bean Chili (page 133).

How to Read Recipes

Reading a recipe is the most important part of cooking. Prior to starting, read through the recipe once to familiarize yourself with it. Then read through it again to assess how much time you will need, what ingredients are required, and if you are familiar with all the terms and techniques. I like to gather my ingredients and tools during this read-through to make sure I have everything needed.

You will read the recipe again as you make your meal. Keep rereading from the top, just to avoid skipping an ingredient or adding the wrong amount of something. Reading and rereading can save you from recipe disaster in the end.

Another thing I have learned as I have cooked is to trust your gut. The more you cook, the more you'll know what looks right and what doesn't. Here is what to look for when reading a recipe:

Title: This is the name of the recipe.

Prep time: This is the approximate time it will take to prepare the ingredients (chopping, dicing, etc.).

Cook time: This is the approximate time needed to cook the recipe.

Headnote: This is the introduction to the recipe.

Yield: This is the amount the recipe will make or how many it will serve.

Ingredient List: This is the list of ingredients needed to make the recipe, typically listed in the order they are used in the recipe.

Directions: These are the step-by-step instructions for making the recipe.

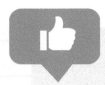

FUN WITH COOKERS

There are a few small kitchen appliances that can make cooking much more efficient but are not necessities. While they may not be allowed in some dorms, you may find them in the common area for your use (or you can bring your own and use them in common areas). They are great for cooking for a group and require little prep work or oversight.

Rice cookers can cook rice perfectly as well as steam vegetables. This small appliance allows you to add the ingredients without having to stir, rotate, or do anything until it's done. Most rice cookers switch automatically to a "keep warm" setting when they are finished.

Slow cookers are great for soups and casseroles. They cook the food slowly without the need for human intervention. In other words, you can start making dinner—just throw all of the ingredients in the cooker—before classes and come back home to a finished meal. I have included a recipe for Slow Cooker Barbecue Sandwiches (page 126). You'll have time to study and still bring the main dish.

The **electric pressure cooker** is what I use most frequently. It enables food to be cooked in about half the time as doing it the traditional way. You can even cook frozen meats (useful if you forgot to defrost before you left for the day) and dried beans. Most electric pressure cookers are catchalls, meaning they can also be used as a yogurt maker, rice cooker, slow cooker, porridge maker, and more.

Cooking Off Book

Although this book contains plenty of recipes to suit a variety of moods and cravings, you may feel inspired to use some of your newly gained cooking knowledge to make something original, which I highly encourage.

On the next page are some things I have learned in my cooking journey that can help you when cooking "off book."

Season: Use seasoning as you cook. Taste as you go, and remember that salt is not a flavor but is used to bring out the flavors of foods.

Acids and Fats: Acids like citrus juices, vinegars, and tomatoes can brighten a dish. Pair them with fats like butter, bacon fat, olive oil, or canola oil to complement the acid and add creaminess to the dish. Marinades are typically one part fat to one part acid, and salad dressings are two parts fat to one part acid.

Mimic What You Know: Use a favorite recipe and flavors as a template to create your own. My mom has this superpower where she can taste every ingredient in a dish and then replicate it. Most of us do not have this talent, so we start with what we know and build on it.

Keep Notes on Your Recipes so You Can Improve on Them: I once made a version of the same casserole seven times before I decided it was perfect. I experimented with herbs and spices, thicker sauce, thinner sauce, cooking times, and adding different flavors.

Experiment with Substitutes: My husband loves chicken salad but not mayonnaise, so we use creamy Caesar salad dressing instead.

Proteins: You can use protein in many ways. Take chicken: One chicken breast has so many meal options. You can shred it and add some taco seasoning for fajitas or taco salad for dinner one night, and then dice it and add it to Alfredo sauce or soup the next. The same is true of plant-based proteins like beans. Drain and rinse a can and add some to a salad or soup for lunch. Make a dip with them for a snack. Then, mash them and spread them on tortillas for dinner.

FIRING UP THE GRILL

Grilling is a great way to cook if you have access to a grill—perfect for a party or tailgate. The grill is so versatile; you can grill fruit, vegetables, and meats. Have you ever tried grilled pineapple? And, of course, there are the tried-and-true grilled items like burgers, hot dogs, steaks, and skewers. This cookbook has a recipe for Grilled Burgers (page 123), and Foil-Baked Chicken (page 77) also comes out delicious on a grill. Flaky fish like cod or halibut is too delicate to cook directly on the grill, but you can cook them in an aluminum foil pouch on the grill. Do not put sugary foods on the grill, as the sugars can cause your food to burn easily.

There are two primary types of grills: gas and charcoal. Grill masters debate which one is better. A gas grill is faster and easier to use, requiring little effort to start and little cleanup. Some say that food grilled over a gas grill isn't as flavorful or takes on a strange taste from the gas. A charcoal grill, on the other hand, does require some preparation. The charcoal needs time to heat up and requires spreading (see Charcoal Grilling Tips on the next page) according to what you're cooking. It also requires more cleanup. But proponents of the charcoal grill prefer the more authentic grilled taste of charcoal-grilled foods.

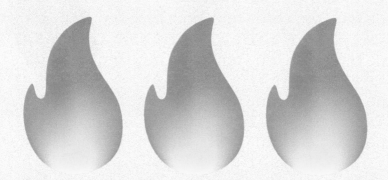

Tips for Grilling on Both Types of Grill:

→ Start with a clean, hot grill.

→ Wipe a little oil on the grilling surface to prevent sticking. I use a pastry brush or paper towel.

→ Frequent turning of grilled items *increases* cooking time.

→ Keep the lid closed as much as possible.

→ Long grilling tongs reduce skin burns.

→ Do not crowd the grill. Instead, cook foods in batches for more even cooking.

→ Use a spoon to place a "dimple" in the top of a burger before grilling. This helps the burger cook evenly and prevents it from inflating.

→ If you're making kebabs with wooden sticks, soak the sticks in water for 30 minutes before grilling. Put similar items on the kebab—things that have similar cooking times.

→ Grilled meat should rest for at least 5 minutes before slicing.

Charcoal Grilling Tips:

→ Stack your charcoal and light it. Allow the coals 15 to 20 minutes to get hot before you begin grilling.

→ Once your coals are hot, spread three-quarters of the coals on one side of the grill to cook hardy meats and one-quarter of the coals on the other side to cook vegetables or more delicate meats like fish.

→ Utilize your vents. The more open the vents, the hotter the coals. Closed vents will put out the coals.

A Note About Safety

Cooking is a wonderful thing, but there are safety concerns to keep in mind.

Fires: Fire is a common kitchen hazard. Never leave anything unattended on the stove. Do not use water on a grease fire. Put it out with baking soda, salt, or a fire extinguisher.

Burns and Splatter: Turn pan handles away from other burners and away from the edge of the stove. Keep oven mitts handy.

Bacteria: Wash your hands before you start cooking and often during the cooking process, especially after handling raw meat. Keep meat, fish, eggs, and dairy refrigerated when not in use. Have two cutting boards—one for meats and one for vegetables and fruit—and wash them immediately with soap and hot water after use. Do not put food on a plate that has had raw meat on it. Make sure to wash fruits and vegetables thoroughly before using.

Knife Safety: A dull knife is a dangerous knife. Always use a sharp knife. Never drop a knife into a sink of dishwater; wash it immediately with warm, soapy water, dry it, and put it away.

Spills: If you spill something, clean it up immediately. Spills can lead to slips and falls in the kitchen or contamination of other foods.

The Recipes in This Book

It's finally time to embark on your college cooking journey. You can always refer back to the list of staple ingredients on page 7, which are the ingredients used most often in this book, and all of the techniques and terms you'll need for these recipes are in this chapter if you need a refresher.

Each recipe in the following chapters indicates any appliances needed, as well as labels to help with menu planning: 15 Minute (for dishes that take 15 minutes or less to prepare from start to finish), Healthy (for dishes that are on the lighter side), No Cook, One Bowl, Vegan, and Vegetarian. The recipes also feature tips on how to reuse ingredients, shop smarter, make a recipe more quickly, make an ingredient from scratch, or cook using a different method in case you don't have the listed appliance. The best way to learn to cook is just to cook, so let's get started.

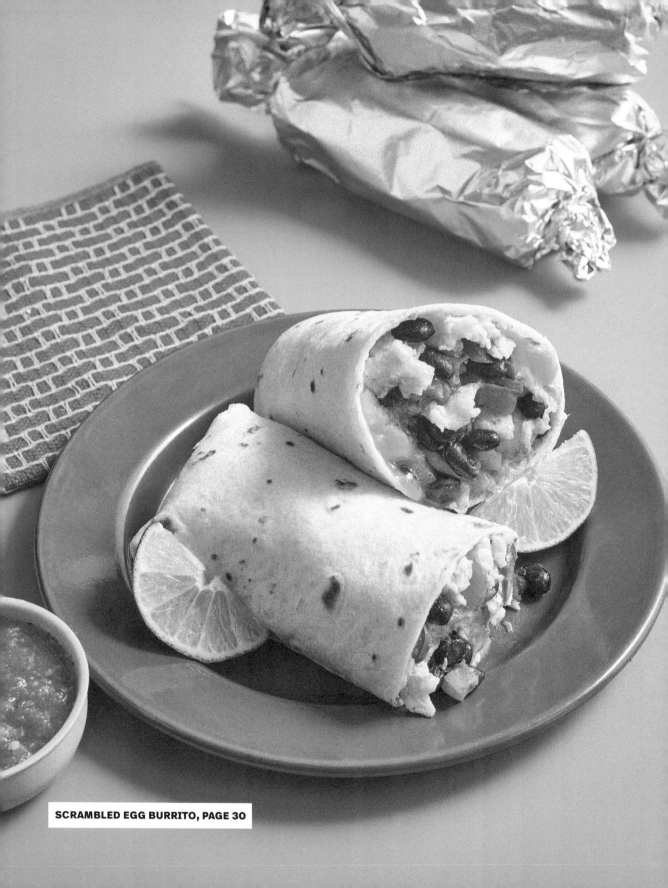

SCRAMBLED EGG BURRITO, PAGE 30

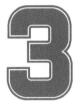

Breakfast

Scrambled Egg Burrito

PREP TIME: 10 minutes **COOK TIME:** 5 minutes **TOTAL TIME:** 15 minutes

Small work space or dorm area? No problem. This scrambled egg burrito requires little preparation and is packed with protein to help fuel you through classes. This recipe can be a foundation for customization: Simply add your favorite burrito ingredients for variety. **SERVES: 1**

Nonstick cooking spray

1 large egg, beaten

¼ cup black beans, drained and rinsed

1 (8-inch) whole-wheat tortilla

½ avocado, mashed (see Guacamole, Smart Shopping Tip, page 46, for how to choose an avocado)

¼ cup plain Greek yogurt

Toppings of your choice (optional), such as grated cheese, break-fast sausage, diced tomatoes, bell peppers, onions, salsa, ketchup, black olives, spinach, or cottage cheese

1. Spray a frying pan with cooking spray and heat over medium heat.

2. Add the egg and beans and cook, stirring continuously, to scramble the egg, about 3 minutes, or until the egg white is no longer runny.

3. Arrange the egg and beans on the tortilla's bottom quarter, and top with mashed avocado and Greek yogurt. Add any other toppings you like (if using). Just be sure not to overstuff your tortilla.

4. Roll the tortilla into a burrito by folding the bottom of the tortilla over the filling. Next, fold one side over about 1 inch. Repeat with the other side (it should look like an open envelope). Now tightly roll the burrito from the bottom until the roll reaches the top of the tortilla.

REMIX TIPS:

→ This is a great way to use up leftovers. Try adding leftover meat (cut into strips or cubes) or leftover vegetables.

→ Skip the tortilla and add the egg to toast with mashed avocado.

Easy French Toast

PREP TIME: 9 minutes **COOK TIME:** 6 minutes **TOTAL TIME:** 15 minutes

This French toast takes so good you won't believe how easy it is to make. Any bread works, but it's especially good with brioche or French bread. Eggs and milk create the custard that makes it so rich. If you can spare the time, and prefer a really custard-y center, let the bread soak in the eggs and milk for longer. **SERVES: 1**

1 large egg

2 tablespoons water

2 tablespoons dairy, nut, or soy milk

¼ teaspoon ground cinnamon (optional)

2 slices bread, each sliced diagonally into 2 triangles

Nonstick cooking spray

Toppings of your choice, such as fresh fruit, maple syrup, powdered sugar, jam, nuts, chocolate chips, coconut, or whipped cream

1. In a small bowl, combine the egg, water, milk, and cinnamon (if using), and whisk until well blended.

2. Dunk the bread triangles in the egg mixture and let them soak for 2 minutes. Flip the bread one time with a spatula to evenly coat and let it soak for another 3 minutes, or until you're ready to start cooking

3. Spray a large frying pan lightly with cooking spray and place over medium heat.

4. Add the soaked bread to the frying pan and cook until golden brown, about 3 minutes. Flip the bread over and cook for another 3 minutes, or until golden brown. Top with your favorite toppings.

REMIX TIPS:

→ Try substituting 2 tablespoons Greek yogurt for the milk to make it a bit tangier. You can also substitute ¼ cup egg substitute for the large egg.

→ Try using cinnamon-raisin bread for a treat.

Avocado Toast

PREP TIME: 5 minutes **COOK TIME:** 3 minutes **TOTAL TIME:** 8 minutes

Avocado toast is not just trendy, it's healthy. Avocado has fiber, healthy fats, and a creamy texture that makes this toast feel indulgent. You can even add an egg for a protein punch. This breakfast (or snack) has so many ways to make it your own: Choose any bread, slice or mash the avocado, and add your favorite seasonings. For a real treat, sprinkle on some coarse salt. **SERVES: 1**

2 slices
  whole-wheat bread

1 avocado, peeled and
  pitted (see Guacamole,
  Smart Shopping Tip,
  page 46, for how to
  choose an avocado)

¼ teaspoon salt

⅛ teaspoon freshly
  ground black pepper

1. Toast the bread to the desired crispiness.

2. Slice the avocado and arrange the slices on the toast, or mash the avocado in a small bowl and then spread it on the toast. Sprinkle with salt and pepper.

REMIX TIPS:

→ You can add 1 teaspoon of lemon juice to the mashed avocado for a fresh, citrusy zing.

→ Try sprinkling ¼ teaspoon red pepper flakes on top to give it a bite.

→ For extra protein, top your toast with an egg, 2 pieces of thinly sliced salmon, or your favorite cheese.

Cottage Cheese and Spinach Scrambled Eggs

PREP TIME: 5 minutes **COOK TIME:** 5 minutes **TOTAL TIME:** 10 minutes

Cottage cheese and spinach scrambled eggs are packed with protein, a combination to fuel your brain. Use any type of cottage cheese, from whole milk to fat-free. This dish was my son Jake's go-to breakfast in college, and when I visit him now, I know this is on his menu for us. **SERVES: 1**

1 tablespoon butter

2 eggs, beaten

¼ cup cottage cheese

¼ teaspoon freshly ground black pepper

1 cup fresh baby spinach

1. Place a small frying pan over medium heat. Put the butter in the pan and allow it to melt.

2. Add the beaten eggs to the pan with the melted butter and cook for 2 minutes, or until they begin to get firm.

3. Add the cottage cheese, pepper, and spinach to the eggs. Using a spatula, begin stirring to break up the eggs and incorporate the cottage cheese. Continue stirring until the spinach wilts and the eggs are set, about 3 minutes.

REMIX TIPS:

→ If you need breakfast to go, transfer the egg mixture to a tortilla and roll it up for a breakfast burrito.

→ Try these add-ins for a flavor change: 2 tablespoons salsa; ¼ cup black beans, drained and rinsed; ¼ cup shredded cheese; 4 tablespoons diced fresh tomato; and/or ⅛ cup diced ham.

Smoothie Bowls Six Ways

PREP TIME: 5 minutes **TOTAL TIME:** 5 minutes

Smoothie bowls are essentially thick, creamy smoothies poured into a bowl and finished with your favorite toppings—such as nuts, seeds, granola, chocolate chips, fresh fruits, and shredded coconut. They resemble ice cream sundaes in flavor and texture more than a little bit. Like sundaes, the flavor combinations are endless. *Unlike* sundaes, they make for a quick, nutritious, and delicious breakfast. Many of these can be made vegan by using nut milks or yogurts. Bonus: If you add a little more liquid and pour it in your to-go cup, you'll have a smoothie to go. **SERVES: 1**

Avocado-Orange Smoothie Bowl

1 small avocado, peeled and pitted (see Guacamole, Smart Shopping Tip, page 46, for how to choose an avocado)

1 banana, peeled and halved

¾ cup orange juice

¼ cup plain Greek yogurt

2 cups ice

Toppings of your choice, such as diced avocado, pumpkin seeds, sunflower seeds, mandarin oranges, pineapple chunks, or shredded coconut

1. In the blender, combine the avocado, banana, juice, yogurt, and ice, and puree until smooth.

2. Pour into a bowl and arrange toppings on top.

Mango and Honey Smoothie Bowl

1 cup frozen mango

¾ cup dairy, nut, or soy milk

1 tablespoon honey

1 (5.3-ounce) container plain Greek yogurt

2 cups ice

Toppings of your choice, such as sunflower seeds, mandarin oranges, pineapple chunks, shredded coconut, or fresh fruit

1. In the blender, combine the mango, milk, honey, yogurt, and ice, and puree until smooth.

2. Pour into a bowl. Add toppings and/or drizzle with more honey.

Banana-Berry Smoothie Bowl

1 banana

¼ cup strawberries, frozen or fresh

¼ cup blueberries, frozen or fresh

¼ cup raspberries, frozen or fresh

1 small apple, cored, peeled, and sliced

¾ cup dairy, nut, or soy milk

Toppings of your choice, such as seeds, fresh berries, sliced bananas, or pineapple chunks

1. In the blender, combine the banana, strawberries, blueberries, raspberries, apple, and milk, and puree until smooth.

2. Pour into a bowl and arrange toppings on top.

CONTINUED »

Green Power Smoothie Bowl

2 celery stalks, chopped

1 small cucumber, peeled and chopped

2 kale leaves

1 cup baby spinach

1 lemon, peeled and sectioned

1 small Granny Smith apple, cored and cut into wedges

2 teaspoons chia seeds

1. In a blender, combine the celery, cucumber, kale, spinach, lemon, apple, and chia seeds, and puree for 1 minute, or until fairly smooth and no large chunks of apple remain.

2. Pour into a bowl and let sit for a few minutes—the longer this smoothie sits, the thicker it will become because of the chia seeds, making it a particularly good choice for a smoothie bowl.

S'mores Snack Smoothie Bowl

1 cup dairy, nut, or soy milk

1 (5.3-ounce) container vanilla Greek yogurt

¾ cup ice

1 tablespoon chocolate syrup

½ cup graham cracker crumbs

¼ cup marshmallow crème or mini marshmallows

1. In the blender, combine the milk, yogurt, and ice, and puree until smooth.

2. Pour into a bowl and top with chocolate syrup, graham cracker crumbs, and marshmallow crème.

Peanut Butter Cup Smoothie Bowl

¾ cup dairy, nut, or soy milk

½ cup creamy
peanut butter

⅓ cup unsweetened
cocoa powder

1 cup ice

2 tablespoons honey

¼ teaspoon salt

Toppings of your choice,
such as seeds, sliced
bananas, chocolate chips,
shredded coconut, peanut
butter, or chocolate syrup

1. In the blender, combine the milk, peanut butter, cocoa powder, ice, honey, and salt, and puree until smooth.

2. Pour into a bowl and arrange toppings on top.

MAKE IT EVEN FASTER TIP: On a 1-quart freezer bag, write the name of the smoothie and the amount of liquid that will need to be added later. Add all of the ingredients (except liquids and yogurt) to the bags and put them in the freezer. When you are ready to make your smoothie, remove the bag of ingredients from the freezer, add it to the blender with liquids and yogurt, and puree.

Microwave Oatmeal

PREP TIME: 2 minutes **COOK TIME:** 3 minutes **TOTAL TIME:** 5 minutes

This is a meal with staying power. After all, the ancient Greeks ate oatmeal. Today, you can microwave this heart-healthy cereal to make a quick breakfast that will keep you satisfied for hours. You can use any type of milk, but make sure to use only old-fashioned oats for this recipe—otherwise your oatmeal will have a mushy texture. **SERVES: 1**

½ cup dairy, nut, or soy milk

½ cup old-fashioned oats

1 teaspoon vanilla extract

¼ teaspoon ground cinnamon

⅛ teaspoon salt

Toppings of your choice, such as peanut butter, seeds, brown sugar, sliced bananas, sliced strawberries, or warm milk

1. In a microwavable bowl, combine the milk, old-fashioned oats, vanilla, cinnamon, and salt. Stir to combine.

2. Place the bowl uncovered in the microwave, and heat on high for 1½ minutes. If you want it softer, try 2 to 2½ minutes.

3. Top with your favorite toppings.

REMIX TIP: You can make overnight oats with no cooking, and just a little planning, for those mornings you need a quick, filling breakfast on the go: In a small mason jar, combine 11 shredded wheat cereal nuggets, 3 tablespoons old-fashioned oats, ¾ cup of your favorite yogurt, 1 tablespoon milk or water, 1 teaspoon honey (optional), ½ cup fresh or frozen berries, and 1 tablespoon nuts (optional). Put the lid on the jar and let it sit in the refrigerator for 6 to 36 hours. When you are ready to eat, stir and enjoy.

Pancakes

PREP TIME: 8 minutes **COOK TIME:** 7 minutes **TOTAL TIME:** 15 minutes

Pretty much every culture has its own type of pancake, from crêpes in France to blini in Russia. So, every college cook needs a go-to pancake recipe. Pancakes are easy to make, and this recipe makes about four pancakes—a perfect single portion. **SERVES: 1**

¼ cup all-purpose flour

1 tablespoon sugar

1 teaspoon
baking powder

⅛ teaspoon salt

1 tablespoon vegetable oil

¼ cup dairy, nut, or
soy milk

1 egg

Nonstick cooking spray

Toppings of your choice
(optional), such as
syrup, jam, jelly, nut
butter, fresh fruit, or
powdered sugar

1. In a medium mixing bowl, combine the flour, sugar, baking powder, and salt. Stir to combine. Make a small well in the dry ingredients.

2. In a small mixing bowl, combine the oil, milk, and egg. Whisk briskly until combined.

3. Pour the wet ingredients into the well in the dry ingredients and mix just until everything is incorporated, making sure there are no big lumps of dry ingredients.

4. Spray a large frying pan with cooking spray and place over medium heat. Let warm for 2 minutes. Using a large spoon or ladle, pour the batter into a 4-inch "puddle" in the pan. You may do this as many times as you can in the pan without the pancakes touching.

5. Let the pancakes cook until bubbles form on the surface, about 3 minutes. Using a spatula, gently flip the pancakes over in the pan and cook until golden brown, about 2 minutes more. Serve with your favorite toppings, if desired.

REMIX TIP: For buttermilk pancakes, add 1 tablespoon white vinegar to ¼ cup regular whole milk and allow to sit for 5 minutes; it will become "lumpy" as it converts to buttermilk. Then, use this buttermilk in place of the milk.

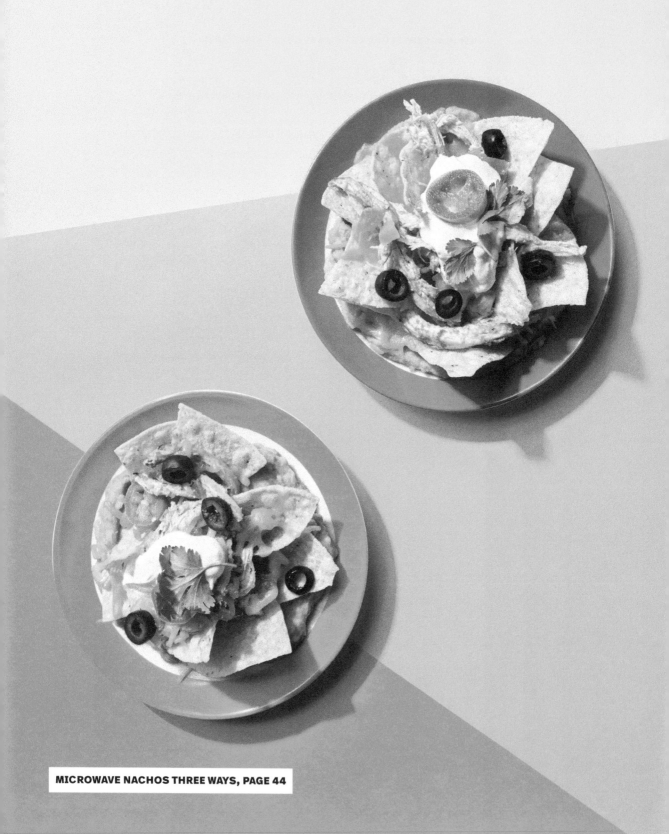

MICROWAVE NACHOS THREE WAYS, PAGE 44

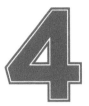

Small Bites and Midnight Snacks

Cheddar Apples

PREP TIME: 3 minutes **COOK TIME:** 2 minutes **TOTAL TIME:** 5 minutes

The combination of apples and cheddar cheese creates a perfect harmony of sweet and savory. You can vary the flavor with different apples (I personally love Gala or Granny Smith). This is an easy, quick snack full of fiber and protein that will keep you full so you can focus on the books.

SERVES: 1

Nonstick cooking spray

1 small apple, cored and
  cut into wedges

⅓ cup grated
  cheddar cheese

1. Preheat the oven to broil. Place a 6-inch piece of foil on a baking sheet and lightly spray with cooking spray.

2. Place the apple wedges on the foil and sprinkle the cheese evenly over the top.

3. Place on the top rack in the oven and heat just until cheese melts, about 2 minutes.

REMIX TIPS:

→ Try adding raisins or chopped walnuts to the top of the apple slices before sprinkling with the cheese.

→ Give it flair by sprinkling on sugar and cinnamon to taste.

→ Experiment with different cheeses, like provolone or Colby.

Microwave Potato Wedges

PREP TIME: 7 minutes **COOK TIME:** 8 minutes **TOTAL TIME:** 15 minutes

These potato wedges are an easy snack or side dish made in the micro-wave in mere minutes—and much better for you than grabbing fries from the fast-food place around the corner. They taste like a baked potato, but you can create new flavor profiles with toppings like cheese, sour cream and chives, and chili, or just keep it simple with ketchup. I highly recommend sprinkling them with 1 teaspoon of grated Parmesan cheese or coarse salt immediately out of the microwave. **SERVES: 1**

2 teaspoons
   Italian dressing

⅛ teaspoon salt

1 medium potato

1. On a microwave-safe plate, combine the Italian dressing and salt.

2. Cut the unpeeled potato lengthwise in half. Cut each half in half again. Now take each quarter and, from the flesh side of the quarter, slice down to create a wedge. This should create 8 wedges.

3. Roll the potato wedges in the Italian dressing mixture until all sides are coated, and arrange the wedges on the plate.

4. Cover the potato wedges with a paper towel and cook in the microwave on high for 4 minutes.

5. Uncover and turn the potato wedges over.

6. Re-cover and cook on high for an additional 4 minutes, or until tender.

REMIX TIP: You can slice any leftovers into small pieces and add them to scrambled eggs, omelets, or soups.

APPLIANCE SWITCH-UP TIP: To make this in a conven-tional oven, bake the seasoned wedges at 425° F for 25 minutes in an uncovered 8-by-8-inch baking dish.

Microwave Nachos Three Ways

PREP TIME: 4 minutes **COOK TIME:** 1 minute **TOTAL TIME:** 5 minutes

These nachos are the perfect snack companion for sitting down to study, and an easy snack to offer when entertaining. They are versatile so you can make them as plain or as dressed up as you like. You can even make this into a full-on meal by adding some leftover chicken or beef. **SERVES: 1**

20 tortilla chips

1½ cups shredded cheese (cheddar, Monterey Jack, or Pepper Jack are all good), divided

1 tablespoon taco seasoning, divided

Additional toppings of your choice (optional), such as black olives, sour cream, salsa, and jalapeños or other green chiles

1. Arrange 10 tortilla chips on a microwave-safe plate. Sprinkle with ½ cup of cheese and ½ tablespoon of taco seasoning.

2. Place in the microwave and heat on high until the cheese melts, about 30 seconds.

3. Add half of the additional toppings you've chosen (if using), then the remaining 10 tortilla chips. Sprinkle with the remaining ½ tablespoon of taco seasoning, 1 cup of cheese, and additional toppings, and microwave on high for 1 minute, or until the cheese melts.

Bean Nachos

20 tortilla chips

½ cup bean dip

1½ cups shredded Monterey Jack cheese

Dip each tortilla chip in bean dip as you place it on a microwave-safe plate. Cover the chips and bean dip with shredded cheese. Microwave on high until the cheese melts and the bean dip is warm, about 2 minutes.

Salsa Nachos

20 tortilla chips

½ cup salsa

1½ cups shredded cheddar, Monterey Jack, or Pepper Jack cheese

Dip each tortilla chip in salsa as you place it on a microwave-safe plate. Sprinkle cheese over the salsa and chips. Microwave on high until the cheese melts, about 1½ minutes.

REMIX TIP: Oh, there are so many options when it comes to nachos. Try these or make them your own. For the best melt, use block cheese and grate it yourself.

Guacamole

PREP TIME: 5 minutes **TOTAL TIME:** 5 minutes

Who doesn't like this universal party dip? Break out the veggie sticks or tortilla chips, whip up a bowl of this easy guacamole, and get to snacking. Make it chunky or smooth; it's totally up to you. If cilantro's not your thing, just delete it or check out the Remix Tips below. **SERVES: 1**

1 large ripe avocado, peeled and pitted (see the Smart Shopping Tip for how to choose an avocado)

2 tablespoons finely chopped fresh cilantro

2 tablespoons finely chopped white onion

1 teaspoon lime juice

¼ teaspoon salt

1. In a small bowl, combine the avocado, cilantro, onion, lime juice, and salt.

2. With a fork, begin mashing the avocado until all ingredients are combined and the texture is how you like it. If you prefer it chunky, try mashing only half the avocado until almost smooth and then folding the other half of the avocado, diced, into the mashed mixture.

3. To store, lay a piece of plastic wrap directly on top of the guacamole, making sure the plastic wrap touches the entire surface (this will keep it from turning brown), and then place in an airtight container in the refrigerator.

REMIX TIP: For a twist, add in 1 tablespoon of your favorite salsa, ¼ teaspoon red pepper flakes, 1 tablespoon blue cheese crumbles, ⅛ teaspoon ground cumin for depth of flavor, or ⅛ teaspoon finely minced garlic.

SMART SHOPPING TIP: When choosing an avocado, you'll want to think about when you plan to eat it. If it is for immediate use (the next 24 hours), select the avocado by using your thumb to applying pressure to the avocado. If it is firm, not mushy and not hard, and allows your thumb to indent the avocado, it is ripe and ready.

MAKE IT FASTER TIP: If you have unripe avocados and want to use them in the next 48 hours, place them in a brown paper bag with a banana.

Cheese Ball
PREP TIME: 14 minutes **COOK TIME:** 6 minutes **TOTAL TIME:** 20 minutes

This cheese ball is a filling, easy-to-make treat that pairs nicely with sliced apples, pears, crackers, and pretzels. It can even be used as a bagel spread. It is a snack that you can store in the refrigerator for up to two weeks. For a firmer cheese ball, wrap it in plastic wrap and place in the refrigerator for at least 45 minutes before eating. **SERVES: 1**

½ cup (about 3 ounces) regular cream cheese

¼ cup butter, softened

1 teaspoon Worcestershire sauce

½ teaspoon onion powder

½ teaspoon garlic powder

3 cups grated cheddar cheese

½ cup finely chopped nuts (optional)

1. Put the cream cheese in a medium microwave-safe bowl and microwave on high for 15 seconds, or until the cheese softens.

2. To the cream cheese in the bowl, add the butter, Worcestershire sauce, onion powder, and garlic powder. Stir in the cheddar cheese and microwave on low for 5 minutes.

3. Put the mixture in a blender (or use a hand mixer if you have one) and blend for 30 seconds. Scrape the mixture out of the blender and onto wax paper or back into the bowl.

4. Use your hands to shape the mixture into a ball.

5. Roll in the chopped nuts (if using) to make a flavorful "crust."

REMIX TIPS:

→ To switch up the flavor, try rolling the cheese ball in these instead of the chopped nuts: ½ cup bacon crumbs, ½ cup cracker crumbs, ½ cup seeds (pumpkin, sunflower, sesame), or ½ cup crushed tortilla chips.

→ Save the broken crackers and chips from the bottom of the bag and crush them to make a great crust for your cheese ball!

→ Try replacing the cheddar cheese with another favorite cheese, like Swiss or Gouda.

Pizza Melt

PREP TIME: 7 minutes   **COOK TIME:** 8 minutes   **TOTAL TIME:** 15 minutes

What's better than a traditional grilled cheese sandwich? A grilled cheese sandwich that brings pizza into the mix! Comfort food times two. Use the recipe as a basic guide, and then feel free to add your favorite pizza toppings, keeping in mind that less is more when it comes to the amount of each ingredient. **SERVES: 1**

1½ tablespoons butter

2 slices bread

2 slices cheddar cheese

5 slices pepperoni

2 teaspoons pizza sauce
  (or marinara)

1. Generously butter one side of each slice of bread. Place a medium skillet over medium heat and let warm for 2 minutes. Place one slice of the buttered bread in the skillet, butter-side down. Top with one slice of cheese and the pepperoni slices. Add the pizza sauce and spread it evenly. Place a second slice of cheese on top of the sauce, and then the second slice of bread, butter-side up. Cook for 4 minutes, or until a light golden brown on the bottom.

2. Using a spatula, flip the sandwich over. Cook for 4 minutes more, or until the second side is a light golden brown and the cheese has melted.

REMIX TIP: Switch it up with your favorite pizza toppings. Think spinach, shredded chicken, a white pizza sauce, ground beef, sausage crumbles, or sliced black olives.

Charcuterie Board

PREP TIME: 10 minutes **TOTAL TIME:** 10 minutes

A charcuterie board looks as impressive as its name sounds, even though it's really just a fancy way of saying a platter of sliced meats, cheeses, fruits, and condiments. This easy-to-eat finger food makes a perfect snack for a lone study session or for a gathering of your friends. It has loads of protein, can be made in a few minutes, and offers a variety of flavors and textures. The list of ingredients below is merely a guide; you should tailor it to your own taste. **SERVES: 1**

6 crackers

4 slices salami

4 slices pepperoni

¼ cup cubed cheese, like cheddar, Swiss, provolone, or Monterey Jack

4 slices of your favorite cheese

2 pickle spears

4 green olives stuffed with pimentos

4 black olives

½ cup red grapes

1 small apple, sliced thinly or in wedges

1 tablespoon nut butter

On a plate or cutting board, lay out all your ingredients (see Make It Yourself Tips below). Serve and enjoy.

MAKE IT YOURSELF TIPS:

→ When making a charcuterie board, it is best to place larger items, like meats and cheese, first. Then use smaller items (bread and crackers), daintier finger foods (like fruits), and jams to fill in the gaps.

→ You can place everything on your board ahead of time, except the crackers and bread, cover with aluminum foil, and place in the refrigerator. Just before serving, add bread and crackers.

→ If you are creating a charcuterie board for a group, think of your board as a mirror: Make sure each half of the board has a bit of everything, so people don't have to reach to get to an item.

REMIX TIP: Try one of these "theme" boards for some extra fun.

→ Pizza: crackers, your favorite sauces, cheeses, olives, and pepperoni

→ Dessert: chocolates, nut butter, and bite-size brownies, cookies, and cakes

→ Nutty: various nut butters and an assortment of nuts

Cheese Quesadilla

PREP TIME: 10 minutes **COOK TIME:** 5 minutes **TOTAL TIME:** 15 minutes

This cheese quesadilla combines the ooey-gooey goodness of a crispy outer crust with a melt-in-your-mouth cheese combo in the center. It is quick to make, packed with protein, and versatile—add beans, salsa, chicken, steak, vegetables, or pepperoni to satisfy your cravings. Use a pizza cutter to cut into perfect triangles for dipping. **SERVES: 1**

Nonstick cooking spray

⅓ cup cream cheese

2 (8-inch) flour tortillas

½ cup shredded cheddar cheese

½ cup shredded Monterey Jack cheese

⅓ cup shredded Pepper Jack cheese

Toppings of your choice (optional): sour cream, Guacamole (page 46), Easy Salsa (page 159), onions, or olives

APPLIANCE SWITCH-UP

TIP: To make these quesadillas in the microwave, spread cream cheese evenly over one side of each tortilla. Place one tortilla on a microwave-safe plate. Add the shredded cheese and top with the second tortilla. Put in the microwave and heat on high for 1 minute.

1. Spray a medium frying pan with cooking spray and place over medium-high heat. Let warm for 1 minute.

2. Using a butter knife, spread the cream cheese evenly over one side of each tortilla.

3. Lay one tortilla in the pan faceup and sprinkle with the shredded cheeses. Add the second tortilla facedown on top of the cheese.

4. Cook for 3 minutes, or until the cheese melts. Lift the edge of the quesadilla and, if that side is golden, use a spatula to flip the tortilla over. Cook another 2 minutes, or until the other side is golden brown. Cut into triangles and serve with the toppings of your choice, if desired.

REMIX TIPS:

→ For a bean and cheese quesadilla, add 2 tablespoons refried beans to the bottom tortilla. Spread the beans evenly over the cream cheese, then sprinkle with shredded cheese.

→ For a chicken and cheese quesadilla, add ¼ cup cubed or shredded cooked chicken on top of the cheese before covering with the second tortilla.

Toaster Oven Caramelized Bacon

PREP TIME: 5 minutes **COOK TIME:** 15 minutes **TOTAL TIME:** 20 minutes

Wake your roommates with the aroma of bacon crisping. Using your toaster oven, you can make six pieces of bacon to your liking, whether you prefer bendy and limp or firm and crisp. If you're planning on using the bacon as a side for eggs, start the bacon first in the toaster oven, and it will be close to finished when your eggs are ready. For a protein-packed snack, try bacon and peanut butter. **SERVES: 1**

6 thick-cut bacon slices

1 tablespoon brown sugar

1. Line the toaster oven tray with aluminum foil. Preheat the toaster oven to 400°F.

2. Lay the bacon slices flat on the foil and sprinkle with brown sugar. Place the bacon in the toaster oven and bake for 12 to 15 minutes, depending on how crispy you like your bacon.

3. Remove the bacon from the toaster oven and put it on a plate lined with a paper towel. Let rest for 1 minute before enjoying.

REMIX TIP: Make it spicy by replacing the plain brown sugar with a mixture of ½ teaspoon cayenne pepper, 1 teaspoon red pepper flakes, 1 teaspoon freshly ground black pepper, and ⅓ cup packed light brown sugar.

MAKE IT EVEN FASTER TIP: For traditional bacon, use the microwave instead by placing 3 paper towels on a microwave-safe plate, laying the bacon strips flat on the paper towels, and covering the bacon with 2 more paper towels. Microwave on high for 4 minutes or 6 minutes for crispy bacon.

Mozzarella Sticks

PREP TIME: 10 minutes **COOK TIME:** 15 minutes **TOTAL TIME:** 25 minutes

So simple, yet so delicious. And this version is even healthier than the restaurant appetizer version because it's baked rather than deep-fried. Make up a batch or two when you're hosting study sessions, bring them to game-day parties, or just have them around so that you can indulge in a few when the midnight cravings come calling. **MAKES: 16 STICKS**

8 (1-ounce) string cheese sticks, halved crosswise

1 egg, whisked

1 cup herbed bread crumbs

1 cup marinara sauce

1. Preheat the oven to 425°F. Line a rimmed baking sheet with parchment paper.

2. Dip each of the string cheese pieces into the egg and shake off any excess. Roll in the bread crumbs to coat and arrange them on the baking sheet so that the pieces are not touching.

3. Bake for 15 minutes, or until the cheese is beginning to melt and the bread crumbs are lightly browned.

4. Serve with the marinara sauce for dipping.

REMIX TIP: Mix 1 tablespoon grated Parmesan cheese into the bread crumbs.

Corn Fritters

PREP TIME: 14 minutes **COOK TIME:** 6 minutes **TOTAL TIME:** 20 minutes

These fritters fare well as a snack or a side dish. They are basically a showcase for sweet corn. You can use fresh, frozen, or canned corn for this recipe. You can top them with sour cream or, for traditionalists, with maple syrup like they do in the South. **SERVES: 1**

¾ cup corn kernels, thawed if frozen, drained if canned

1 scallion, white and light green parts only, sliced

¼ cup all-purpose flour

¼ teaspoon salt

2 tablespoons nut or soy milk

1 tablespoon extra-virgin olive oil, plus more as needed

1. In a large bowl, stir together the corn, scallion, flour, and salt. Stir in the milk. The mixture should be pretty thick and just barely sticking together. Form it into two loose patties.

2. In a large skillet over medium heat, heat the olive oil. Once the oil is hot (test by flicking some water off your fingers into the skillet; it should sizzle), add the fritters and cook for 2 to 3 minutes, or until browned. Flip and cook for 2 to 3 minutes more, adding more oil as needed.

REMIX TIPS:

→ Stir in 1 teaspoon diced jalapeño, ½ teaspoon lime juice, and 1 tablespoon chopped fresh cilantro.

→ For even more deliciousness, add 2 tablespoons grated cheddar cheese.

Chocolate Milkshake

PREP TIME: 5 minutes **TOTAL TIME:** 5 minutes

If you learn to make just one thing in the blender, it should be this: a chocolate milkshake. Nothing could be easier, and once you have the method down, you can add your own twist. It's such a simple indulgence, but it'll "shake" up your world (or at least make a night of studying a whole lot better). **SERVES: 1**

1 cup chocolate ice cream

¼ cup half-and-half or whole milk

1. In a blender, combine the ice cream and half-and-half.

2. Blend with the lid on for 1 minute, or until smooth.

REMIX TIPS:

→ Add 1 tablespoon chocolate syrup for an extra rich chocolate milkshake, or substitute your favorite ice cream flavor to create a different flavor milkshake.

→ Try these varieties: For *cookies and cream*, add three chocolate sandwich cookies with the ice cream. For *brownie*, cut 1 brownie into small squares and add to the blender once your milkshake is made, then "pulse" a few times to distribute the brownie into the shake. For *double chocolate*, after the milkshake is made, add 2 tablespoons mini-chocolate chips and stir by hand to distribute.

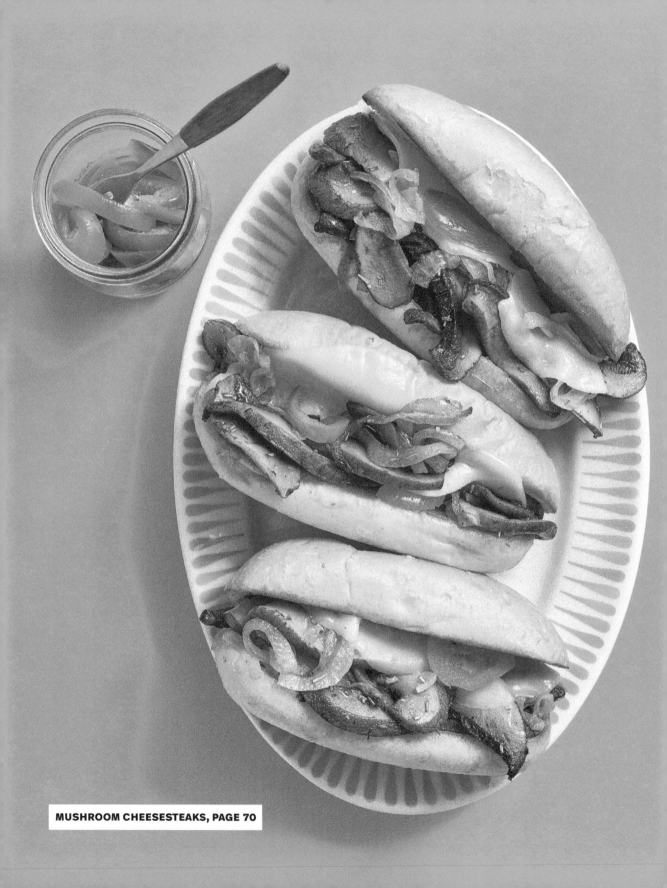

MUSHROOM CHEESESTEAKS, PAGE 70

5

To-Go Food

Easy Chicken Salad

PREP TIME: 5 minutes **COOK TIME:** 5 minutes **TOTAL TIME:** 10 minutes

For a protein boost packed with nutrients from the fruits and veggies, make this easy microwave chicken salad—it will quickly become a staple in your lunch repertoire. Make ahead for snacking, packing, and eating on the go in a tortilla wrap, on salad greens, or with crackers. **SERVES: 1**

1 medium boneless,
  skinless chicken breast

⅓ cup diced celery

⅓ cup seedless green
  grapes, halved

⅓ cup seedless red
  grapes, halved

1 tablespoon
  sliced scallions

⅓ cup chopped
  walnuts (optional)

¼ cup mayonnaise

1 teaspoon Dijon mustard

⅛ teaspoon salt

⅛ teaspoon freshly
  ground black pepper

1. Place the chicken breast in an 8-by-8-inch microwave-safe dish and fill with water until water is one-third the depth of the chicken.

2. Cover the dish with plastic wrap and cook on high for 4 to 5 minutes. Use a meat thermometer to check that the internal temperature has reached 165°F.

3. Allow the chicken to cool for 5 minutes, then dice or shred it.

4. In a medium bowl, combine the chicken, celery, grapes, scallions, and walnuts (if using). Toss to break up and evenly disperse ingredients.

5. Add the mayonnaise, mustard, salt, and pepper and mix well.

6. Cover and refrigerate until ready to go. To make as a wrap, scoop chicken salad onto a tortilla and fold into a burrito shape (see page 30). Wrap the bottom with a paper towel and be on your way!

REMIX TIP: You can substitute Caesar dressing for the mayonnaise, or try using 2 to 3 tablespoons of hummus. To make it vegan, substitute ¾ cup canned black-eyed peas, drained and rinsed, for the chicken and 2 to 3 tablespoons of hummus for the mayonnaise.

Turkey Salad Pita

PREP TIME: 5 minutes **COOK TIME:** 2 minutes **TOTAL TIME:** 7 minutes

This turkey salad is colorful and tasty. It uses sliced deli meat rather than the traditional "flaked" meat. But you can always lift some leftovers from Thanksgiving break and use that instead. To avoid sogginess, don't fill the pita pockets until you are ready to eat. **SERVES: 1**

1 cup baby spinach

½ cup thinly sliced red bell pepper

6 tablespoons mayonnaise

3 ounces sliced cooked deli turkey

½ avocado, pitted, peeled, and diced (see Guacamole, Smart Shopping Tip, page 46, for how to choose an avocado)

½ tablespoon sunflower seeds

¼ teaspoon salt

⅛ teaspoon freshly ground black pepper

1 whole-wheat pita

1. Preheat the toaster oven to broil.

2. In a large bowl, combine the spinach, red bell pepper, and mayonnaise, and lightly toss to coat the spinach with mayonnaise.

3. Add the turkey, avocado, and sunflower seeds, and season with salt and pepper.

4. Put the pita under the broiler for 1 minute. Gently turn over and cook for 1 minute on the other side. Do not brown the pita.

5. Cut the pita in half and gently separate each half to create two "pockets." Fill each with the turkey salad. Wrap the pita pockets in a paper towel so they are easier to hold and you don't drop any of the filling.

REMIX TIPS:

→ Replace the mayonnaise with hummus or creamy Caesar dressing.

→ Substitute marinated pimento slices for the red bell pepper. Or try adding halved cherry tomatoes or olive slices.

→ Replace turkey with your favorite deli meat: Roast beef, chicken, or ham all work well.

MAKE IT EVEN FASTER: Make a no-cook version by using a whole-wheat tortilla or whole-wheat bread.

Cobb Salad

PREP TIME: 15 minutes **COOK TIME:** 20 minutes **TOTAL TIME:** 35 minutes

The Cobb salad is a meal salad. The toppings for this salad make a fun acronym with the name of the salad, so "EAT COBB": Egg, Avocado, Tomato, Chicken, Onion, Bacon, and Blue cheese. It all comes together with a bright vinaigrette dressing. This may be a good one to try on a weekend because it does require a bit of prep time. Nothing difficult, though. Start by hard-boiling the egg (while you've got the water boiling, consider hard-boiling some extras so you have them for other dishes), and cooking the bacon and the chicken, in that order. Note, a 3- to 4-ounce chicken breast is about the size of a deck of playing cards.

SERVES: 1

1 large egg

1 (3- to 4-ounce) boneless, skinless chicken breast

¾ teaspoon salt

½ teaspoon freshly ground black pepper

⅛ teaspoon paprika

2 bacon slices

1 cup romaine lettuce, cut into ½-inch strips (about half a medium head)

5 cherry tomatoes, halved

1. In a small saucepan, cover the egg with cold water by 1 inch. Bring the water to a boil over medium-high heat, then turn off the heat and cover. Let sit for 10 minutes. Meanwhile, fill a bowl with ice water. Using a slotted spoon, transfer the egg to the bowl of ice water. Let sit for 5 minutes, then peel and slice.

2. While the egg is boiling, season the chicken with salt, pepper, and paprika. Put the chicken breast in an 8-by-8-inch microwave-safe dish and fill with water until water is one-third the depth of the chicken.

3. Cover the dish with plastic wrap and cook on high for 4 to 5 minutes. Use a meat thermometer to check that the internal temperature has reached 165°F.

4. Allow the chicken to cool for 5 minutes before dicing it into ½-inch pieces.

1 avocado, peeled, pitted, and diced (see Guacamole, Smart Shopping Tip, page 46, for how to choose an avocado)

¼ cup finely chopped onion

2 tablespoons crumbled blue cheese

⅛ cup Basic Vinaigrette (page 164)

5. While the chicken is cooling, line a microwave-safe plate with three paper towels. Add the bacon, top with three more paper towels, and microwave on high for 3 minutes. Turn bacon over and microwave on high for 3 minutes more. If you want your bacon crispier, microwave in increments of 30 seconds to reach the desired texture.

6. In a 1-quart mason jar, bowl, or resealable container, layer the salad in this order: lettuce, tomatoes, avocado, onion, blue cheese, chicken, bacon, and egg.

7. When ready to eat, drizzle the vinaigrette over salad.

REMIX TIPS:

→ Substitute ham or turkey for the chicken.

→ To make it vegetarian, use ¾ cup canned black-eyed peas, drained and rinsed, instead of the chicken, and omit the bacon.

MAKE IT EVEN FASTER: Buy the egg, chicken, and bacon pre-cooked to save time. You can also grab a ready-made vinaigrette dressing to save even more time. You may be able to source these items from the dining hall, if you have a food plan.

Bran Muffins

PREP TIME: 12 minutes **COOK TIME:** 18 minutes **TOTAL TIME:** 30 minutes

Make your own muffins rather than grabbing sugar-filled ones at the campus coffee place. These bran muffins are quick and fun to create, and they make a filling and delicious to-go meal. They may taste like a treat, but they'll keep you fueled and focused for hours. **MAKES: 4 MUFFINS**

½ cup bran cereal

½ cup dairy, nut, or
    soy milk

½ cup all-purpose flour

2 tablespoons sugar

1 teaspoon
    baking powder

¼ teaspoon salt

2 tablespoons
    vegetable oil

Nonstick cooking spray

1. Preheat the oven to 400°F. In a small bowl, combine the bran cereal and milk. Stir to coat the cereal and let sit for 5 minutes.

2. Meanwhile, in another mixing bowl, combine the flour, sugar, baking powder, and salt, and mix to evenly distribute. Make a well in the center.

3. When the cereal has absorbed most of the milk, add the vegetable oil and stir.

4. Pour the cereal mixture into the well in the dry ingredients and stir just until moistened.

5. In four greased muffin-tin cups, or paper muffin liners sprayed with cooking spray, evenly divide the mixture. (Tins or muffin liners should be about halfway full.)

6. Place on the center rack of the oven and bake for 18 minutes, or until a toothpick inserted in the center comes out clean. Let the muffins rest in the tin for 5 minutes before removing them.

7. Never store muffins in the refrigerator. This will dry them out and change their texture. Instead, line an airtight container with a paper towel. Put the muffins in the container and top them with a paper towel before sealing the container. The muffins will stay fresh for up to 3 days.

REMIX TIPS:

→   Stir in dried fruit such as raisins, apricots, or cranberries. Add these in step 2.

→   Add 2 tablespoons semisweet chocolate chips to
the dry mix in step 2.

→   Make an orange glaze and drizzle on the muffins: Whisk together ¼ teaspoon orange juice,
⅛ teaspoon vanilla extract, 2 tablespoons
powdered sugar, and ½ tablespoon milk. If
too thick, add more milk. If too thin, add more
powdered sugar.

APPLIANCE SWITCH-UP: Bake these muffins in the toaster
oven. The cook time may vary greatly, but try baking for
9 to 10 minutes at 400° F to start.

Avocado-Orange Salad

PREP TIME: 10 minutes **TOTAL TIME:** 10 minutes

This easy salad combines creamy, mellow avocado with the bright, zesty flavor of mandarin oranges. It tastes so fresh that it will put a little zing in your step. For even easier preparation, combine the ingredients in a quart-size mason jar and shake vigorously when ready to eat. You'll combine the dressing, coat the salad, and create a to-go cup at the same time. **SERVES: 1**

¼ cup Italian dressing

2 tablespoons
  orange juice

1 tablespoon lime juice

⅛ teaspoon salt

1 cup spring mix or
  coarsely chopped
  romaine lettuce

1 avocado, peeled, pitted,
  and diced (see Guaca-
  mole, Smart Shopping
  Tip, page 46, for how to
  choose an avocado)

1 (11-ounce) can mandarin
  oranges, drained

¼ cup thinly sliced
  red onion

1. In a small jar with a tight-fitting lid, make the dressing by combining the Italian dressing, orange juice, lime juice, and salt. Shake vigorously until well combined and the salt has dissolved.

2. In a quart-size mason jar or resealable container, top the lettuce with the avocado, oranges, and red onion. Drizzle with the dressing and be on your way.

REMIX TIPS:

→ If you'd like to use fresh oranges, use 2 mandarins or 1 small navel orange.

→ These make great additions to the salad in any combination: 1 cup diced cooked chicken; 1 cup fresh raspberries; 3 tablespoons chopped pecans; ¼ cup halved grapes; 2 slices of provolone cheese; a sliced hard-boiled egg; dried fruit.

Salmon and Cucumber Salad

PREP TIME: 10 minutes **TOTAL TIME:** 10 minutes

This salmon and cucumber salad has plenty of omega-3s to keep your brain operating at top performance. This is a go-to lunch on a warm day; it offers a lot of texture and is incredibly easy to make, thanks to the canned salmon. It's also deceptively filling, considering its fresh and light feel. Make it in a mason jar or resealable container to eat between classes or on the go. **SERVES: 1**

½ avocado, pitted, peeled, and mashed (see Guacamole, Smart Shopping Tip, page 46, for how to choose an avocado)

½ green bell pepper, chopped

2 tablespoons finely chopped fresh parsley

2 teaspoons extra-virgin olive oil, divided

1 teaspoon lime juice

1 teaspoon Dijon mustard

⅛ teaspoon salt

⅛ teaspoon freshly ground black pepper

½ cup canned no-salt-added salmon, drained

4 romaine lettuce leaves, chopped

½ cup sliced cucumber

1. In a medium mixing bowl, combine the avocado, bell pepper, parsley, 1 teaspoon of olive oil, the lime juice, mustard, salt, and pepper. Toss lightly.

2. Use a fork to gently flake the salmon in the can, then add it to the avocado mixture.

3. On a plate or in a quart-size mason jar, place the romaine lettuce leaves. Top with the salmon mixture. Add the sliced cucumbers and drizzle with the remaining teaspoon of olive oil.

REMIX TIPS:

→ Try adding your favorite salad dressing or Basic Vinaigrette (page 164) for additional flavor.

→ This easily converts to a wrap: Just lay one whole romaine leaf on the bottom third of a tortilla, top with salmon and cucumbers, and then roll into a wrap. Or eat as a lettuce wrap without the tortilla.

Taco Salad

PREP TIME: 10 to 15 minutes **TOTAL TIME:** 10 to 15 minutes

When you're missing Taco Tuesdays, try this for a quick fix. Add chicken or ground beef if you're not in the mood for this vegetarian version. You can put everything in a quart-size mason jar or resealable dish and take it to go. Just remember to pack the corn chips in a separate container until you're ready to eat to prevent them from getting soggy. No one likes a wet corn chip. **SERVES: 1**

¼ cup salsa

2 tablespoons plain Greek yogurt

1 teaspoon taco seasoning

½ avocado, pitted, peeled and diced (see Guacamole, Smart Shopping Tip, page 46, for how to choose an avocado)

2 hard-boiled eggs, chopped (see Cobb Salad, page 60, for hard-boiling instructions, or buy pre-cooked)

5 cherry tomatoes, halved

⅓ cup black beans, drained and rinsed

1½ cups shredded lettuce

½ cup corn chips

1. In a quart-size mason jar, combine the salsa, yogurt, and taco seasoning. Stir until well mixed.

2. Add the avocado, eggs, tomatoes, beans, and lettuce. Tighten the lid and you're all set.

3. Add corn chips and give the jar a shake when you're ready to eat.

REMIX TIPS:

→ Boost your protein even more by including ¾ cup chopped rotisserie chicken, pre-cooked chicken breast, or cooked ground beef in step 2.

→ Try adding your favorite taco toppings, such as shredded cheddar cheese, diced onions, sliced olives, more salsa, and/or Guacamole (page 46).

Fruit and Yogurt Parfait

PREP TIME: 10 minutes **TOTAL TIME:** 10 minutes

The word "parfait" *perfectly* describes this dessert-like, healthy treat. Make this before bed for a grab-and-go-breakfast or, if you can't resist, enjoy it as a late-night snack. You can swap out the fruit for whatever you have on hand. Fresh or canned fruit both work great. You can make more layers if you like by using less of each ingredient per layer. **SERVES: 1**

1 cup of your
  favorite yogurt

¾ cup sliced fruit of
  your choice, such as
  strawberries, peaches,
  oranges, or bananas

¼ cup Traditional Granola
  (page 162) or store-
  bought granola (optional)

1 tablespoon chopped
  unsalted walnuts
  (optional)

1. In a 10-ounce mason jar, spoon half of the yogurt. Top with half of the fruit and half of the granola and nuts (if using).

2. Add a second layer of yogurt, fruit, granola, and nuts. Put the lid on the jar and head off to class.

REMIX TIPS:

→ Substitute 10 pieces of shredded wheat or nugget cereal for the granola.

→ Try matching yogurt flavors to the fruit, like orange yogurt with mandarin orange slices or peach yogurt with peach slices. Or use the yogurt to complement the fruit, like coconut yogurt with pineapple slices or lemon yogurt with fresh berries.

→ Turn this into a true dessert by adding a dollop of Homemade Whipped Cream (page 165), a few chocolate chips, or a drizzle of honey.

Asparagus Pasta Salad

PREP TIME: 5 minutes   **COOK TIME:** 10 to 20 minutes   **TOTAL TIME:** 15 to 25 minutes

This superb salad travels well and can be tailored to any craving. Three tips for success: Use a pasta that has ridges and curves like penne, spiral, or rotini to help it hold up to the mixing. Always slightly undercook the pasta just a minute less than the full time on the package directions, to keep the pasta from breaking apart or turning mushy in the salad. Finally, wait for the pasta to cool completely before you add it to the other ingredients. **SERVES: 1**

⅓ cup uncooked rotini

3 tablespoons
  Italian dressing

¼ teaspoon
  Dijon mustard

¼ teaspoon minced garlic

½ teaspoon salt

⅛ teaspoon freshly
  ground black pepper

1 small tomato, chopped

¼ cup sliced black olives

1 (15-ounce) can
  extra-long green aspar-
  agus spears, drained
  and chopped

1. Cook the pasta according to the package directions or in a microwave (see Rice and Pasta in the Microwave, page 16). Drain, then rinse under cold water.

2. In a medium bowl, combine the Italian dressing, mustard, garlic, salt, and pepper. Mix until well blended.

3. Add the cooked pasta, tomato, black olives, and asparagus. Toss to coat. Transfer the salad to a mason jar for easy portability.

REMIX TIP: Try adding steamed broccoli florets, diced red and green bell pepper, salami, pepperoni, diced ham, marinated mozzarella balls, or crumbled feta cheese for a twist.

Chocolate-Hazelnut Swirl Banana Muffins

PREP TIME: 10 minutes **COOK TIME:** 15 minutes **TOTAL TIME:** 25 minutes

I developed this recipe in college and still make it to this day. Because my dorm room didn't have an oven, I would make the batter for the muffins in my room and bake them in the communal kitchen's oven. It is a great recipe for when you have a few brown bananas lying around, access to an oven, and some roommates with a sweet tooth. **MAKES: 6 MUFFINS**

Nonstick cooking
  spray (optional)

¾ cup all-purpose flour

¼ teaspoon baking soda

¼ teaspoon
  baking powder

1½ ripe bananas

¼ cup sugar

1 large egg

2 tablespoons
  vegetable oil

1 teaspoon vanilla extract

6 tablespoons
  chocolate-hazelnut
  spread, divided

1. Preheat the oven to 350°F. Line a muffin pan with 6 liners, or place liners on a baking sheet. Spray liners with cooking spray (if using).

2. In a mixing bowl, whisk together the flour, baking soda, and baking powder. Set aside.

3. In a separate bowl, mash the bananas until smooth. Add the sugar, egg, oil, and vanilla. Mix very well.

4. Slowly pour the flour mixture, while whisking, into the banana mixture. Whisk until the mixtures are well combined.

5. Fill the muffin liners until three-quarters full (about 3 tablespoons of batter each). Top each muffin with 1 tablespoon of chocolate-hazelnut spread, and use a toothpick or knife to swirl it into the batter.

6. Bake for 15 to 17 minutes, or until a toothpick inserted in the center comes out clean.

REMIX TIP: If you want to taste more chocolate and hazelnut in your first bite, I would recommend just swirling lightly at the top. If you want the spread to bake more into the muffin, you can use your toothpick to push it deeper.

Mushroom Cheesesteaks

PREP TIME: 5 minutes **COOK TIME:** 15 minutes **TOTAL TIME:** 20 minutes

Let's take a culinary trip to Philly. The traditional cheesesteak is typically made with thin slices of sautéed rib-eye steak and melted cheese placed on a long, crusty roll. This vegetarian take on Philadelphia's classic sandwich incorporates sliced portobello mushrooms, rosemary, and cayenne instead. To boost the flavor even more and add crunch, throw on some pickled veggies of any kind. **MAKES: 2 SANDWICHES**

1 tablespoon vegetable oil

½ onion, thinly sliced

2 fresh portobello mushroom caps, cut into ¼-inch slices

½ teaspoon crushed dried rosemary (optional)

¼ teaspoon cayenne pepper (optional)

¼ teaspoon salt

⅛ teaspoon freshly ground black pepper

2 hoagie rolls, halved

2 provolone cheese slices

1. Preheat the oven to 400°F. Line a baking sheet with parchment paper and set aside.

2. In a large skillet, heat the oil over medium heat. Once the oil is shiny, add the onion and cook for 4 minutes, or until translucent.

3. Add the mushrooms, rosemary (if using), cayenne (if using), salt, and black pepper and cook for 2 minutes, or until the mushrooms begin to darken in color.

4. Arrange the hoagie rolls cut-side up on the lined baking sheet. Evenly divide the mushroom mixture between 2 of the hoagie halves and top with the provolone cheese.

5. Bake until the cheese is melted, about 5 minutes.

6. Place the toasted hoagie halves on top of the mushroom-cheese halves and wrap the sandwiches in foil for a lunch on the go.

REMIX TIP: If you cannot find portobello mushroom caps, swap in 2¼ cups sliced cremini, shiitake, or baby bella mushrooms. Instead of provolone cheese, try Swiss.

Bean-y Burrito Bowl

PREP TIME: 13 minutes **COOK TIME:** 2 minutes **TOTAL TIME:** 15 minutes

Craft this deconstructed burrito with a delicious lime vinaigrette and you'll have a fiesta for one. Use a variety of beans for a boost of protein with minimal effort. A quart-size mason jar allows you to add all ingredients, including the dressing, give it a vigorous shake, and feast. **SERVES: 1**

¼ cup vegetarian refried beans

1½ cups shredded lettuce

½ cup black beans, drained and rinsed

½ cup whole kernel corn

2 tablespoons diced green chiles

3 tablespoons salsa

1 tablespoon extra-virgin olive oil

1 tablespoon lime juice

½ teaspoon garlic powder

½ teaspoon salt

¼ teaspoon ground cumin

¼ teaspoon ground oregano

¼ teaspoon freshly ground black pepper

1. In a microwave-safe bowl, spoon in the refried beans, cover with a damp paper towel, and microwave on high for 1 minute. Stir and cook for 1 more minute. Stir again. If the beans still need to be warmer, microwave them in 30-second intervals, stirring after each.

2. In a mason jar or resealable container, layer the ingredients in this order: lettuce, beans, corn, green chiles, and salsa.

3. In a small bowl, whisk together the olive oil, lime juice, garlic powder, salt, cumin, oregano, and pepper until well combined. Drizzle over the burrito bowl, put on the lid, and give the container a good shake to make sure all the ingredients are well coated with dressing.

REMIX TIP: Other appetizing additions include 1 cup cooked, shredded chicken; ¼ cup rice; 3 tablespoons black olives; ½ avocado, pitted, peeled, and sliced; 5 cherry tomatoes, halved; ¼ pound cooked ground beef; shredded cheddar cheese; and/or a dollop of sour cream.

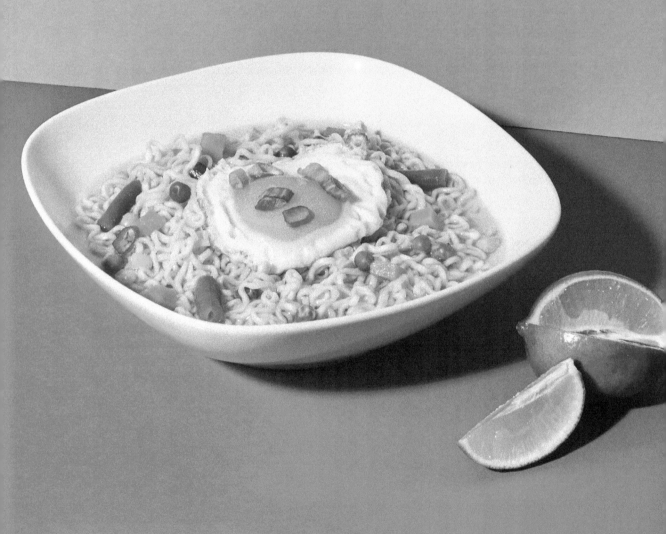

UPGRADED INSTANT RAMEN, PAGE 94

6

Meals for One

Turkey-Stuffed Peppers

PREP TIME: 10 minutes **COOK TIME:** 20 minutes **TOTAL TIME:** 30 minutes

This self-contained meal has everything you need: vitamins from the peppers, protein from the turkey, rice to help fill you up, and a savory-sweet tomato sauce to top it all off. Plus, it is so easy to make in the microwave. This recipe makes two peppers, but you can freeze one and enjoy it another day (see Remix Tip). **MAKES: 2 PEPPERS**

½ pound ground turkey

1 small onion,
    finely chopped

¼ cup water

1 (8-ounce) can tomato
    sauce, divided

1 tablespoon
    Parmesan cheese

½ teaspoon salt

⅛ teaspoon
    ground oregano

⅛ teaspoon freshly
    ground black pepper

¼ cup uncooked
    instant rice

2 large green or red
    bell peppers

1 teaspoon packed
    brown sugar

4 tablespoons shredded
    cheddar cheese, divided

1. In a 1-quart microwave-safe casserole dish, combine the ground turkey and onion. Microwave on high for 4 minutes, or until the turkey is no longer pink, stirring once during cooking. Drain and discard the grease.

2. Stir in the water, half of the tomato sauce, the Parmesan cheese, salt, oregano, and black pepper. Cover with plastic wrap.

3. Put the dish back in the microwave and cook on high for 3 minutes, or until the mixture bubbles. Stir in the rice and re-cover with plastic wrap. Let rest for about 5 minutes.

4. While the mixture is resting, halve the bell peppers lengthwise. Remove the tops, seeds, and stems. Place the bell pepper halves cut-side up in a large microwave-safe dish.

5. Evenly divide the meat/rice filling among the pepper halves.

6. In a small bowl, combine the remaining tomato sauce and the brown sugar. Stir until evenly combined and the brown sugar has dissolved. Spoon the sauce over the assembled peppers.

7. Cover the dish with plastic wrap and microwave on high for 10 minutes, rotating once. Sprinkle the peppers with cheddar cheese and let rest for 5 minutes before serving.

REMIX TIP: To freeze stuffed peppers, first allow them to cool completely. Wrap each stuffed pepper in plastic wrap, then put in a quart-size resealable freezer bag. To reheat the peppers in the microwave, cook them individually on high for 2 minutes.

SMART SHOPPING TIP: Ground turkey is usually sold in 1-pound packages. You can divide a package in half and store it in freezer bags (write the date and "½ pound ground turkey" on the package). Use the meat within 2 days of defrosting.

Microwave Alfredo with Noodles

PREP TIME: 5 minutes **COOK TIME:** 15 minutes **TOTAL TIME:** 20 minutes

Alfredo sauce is so rich and creamy, you'd think it was complicated to make. In fact, you need only three ingredients: Parmesan cheese, butter, and heavy whipping cream. From there, you can add seasonings and ingredients like chicken, mushrooms, spinach, hot sauce, and more to elevate the flavor. A microwave is all you need. **SERVES: 1**

½ cup egg noodles

1 cup water

½ cup grated
  Parmesan cheese

¼ cup butter, cut
  into cubes

¼ cup heavy
  (whipping) cream

¼ teaspoon garlic powder

½ teaspoon salt

¼ teaspoon freshly
  ground black pepper

1. In a deep microwave-safe bowl, combine the egg noodles and water. Cover and cook on high in the microwave for 5 minutes. Stir. Cover and cook another 5 minutes, or until the noodles are tender. Drain and set aside.

2. In a large microwave-safe bowl, combine the Parmesan cheese, butter, heavy cream, garlic powder, salt, and pepper, and microwave on high for 2 minutes, or until the butter melts. Stir twice during cooking.

3. Add the noodles and stir to coat with sauce. Microwave on medium-high for 2 minutes, or until hot.

REMIX TIPS:

→ Add 1 cup cooked and cubed chicken breast, 1 cup thinly sliced beef, or 1 cup cooked shrimp.

→ Add 4 ounces mushrooms (add to water and noodles in step 1).

→ Add some heat with ¼ teaspoon or more of hot sauce.

Foil-Baked Chicken

PREP TIME: 10 minutes **COOK TIME:** 25 minutes **TOTAL TIME:** 35 minutes

You've heard of a one-man band; well, this is a one-pouch meal. You'll love the ease, the heartiness, and the no-mess cleanup of this baked chicken. No plate needed—eat it right out of the foil. Plus, the foil pack keeps all of the flavors intact. **SERVES: 1**

Nonstick cooking spray

1 small sweet
  potato, sliced

1 carrot, peeled and
  sliced into coins

1 small onion, peeled
  and quartered

½ teaspoon minced garlic

1 small (3-ounce)
  chicken breast

½ teaspoon salt

¼ teaspoon freshly
  ground black pepper

¼ teaspoon paprika

1 tablespoon butter

APPLIANCE SWITCH-UP TIP: Make this in the toaster oven by preheating it to 350°F, following the same directions, and baking for 20 minutes.

1. Preheat the oven to 350°F. Spray a 12-by-12-inch piece of aluminum foil with cooking spray.

2. Put the sweet potato and carrot on the foil, allowing the slices to overlap. Add the onion and garlic on top.

3. Season the raw chicken with salt, pepper, and paprika on both sides, and place it on top of the vegetables. Place the butter on top of the chicken.

4. Close the foil tightly by folding two opposite sides toward the middle, over the chicken. Bring the other two opposite sides of the foil toward the center until the edges meet. Roll these edges down to create a seal.

5. Place the chicken on the top rack of the oven, folded-foil-side up, and bake for 25 minutes. Check the internal temperature of the chicken; it is done when it reaches 165°F.

REMIX TIPS:

→ Try adding zucchini slices, cherry tomatoes, celery, or shredded cheese to the chicken before enclosing it in the foil packet

→ Add 1 tablespoon dry ranch dressing powder to the salt and pepper to season the chicken.

Microwave Sloppy Joes

PREP TIME: 5 minutes **COOK TIME:** 10 minutes **TOTAL TIME:** 15 minutes

It is said that this classic sandwich came to being in the early 20th century when a cook named Joe at an Iowan café added tomato sauce to a loose-meat sandwich, served it, and got rave reviews. If you want a leaner meal, substitute ground turkey for the ground beef, or use extra-lean ground beef. **MAKES: 1 SANDWICH**

¼ pound ground beef

1½ tablespoons finely chopped onion

1½ tablespoons finely chopped celery

2 tablespoons ketchup

1½ teaspoons water

1 teaspoon yellow mustard

½ teaspoon packed brown sugar

⅛ teaspoon salt

⅛ teaspoon chili powder

⅛ teaspoon cayenne pepper (optional)

1 hamburger bun

1. In a 1-quart microwave-safe dish, combine the ground beef, onion, and celery. Microwave on high for 3 minutes, stirring one time during cooking. When done, the ground beef should no longer be pink. Drain the dish and break up the meat.

2. Add the ketchup, water, mustard, brown sugar, salt, chili powder, and cayenne (if using), and stir until well mixed. Cover the dish with plastic wrap and microwave on medium for 4 minutes, or until hot.

3. Spoon the beef mixture onto the bun and try your best to eat it without spilling.

REMIX TIPS:

→ Top with shredded cheese of your choice.

→ To prevent the bun from becoming soggy, lightly toast the bun in a toaster or under the broiler in an oven or toaster oven for 1 minute.

Tofu Vegetable Stir-Fry

PREP TIME: 10 minutes **COOK TIME:** 10 minutes **TOTAL TIME:** 20 minutes

Pull out the chopsticks and dig into this fresh, delicious, quick dish. Boasting all nine essential amino acids, this protein (made from bean curd) has too many health benefits to list here. Marinate the tofu for at least 10 minutes—but the longer it sits, the more flavor it will carry into the dish. **YIELD: 1 SERVING**

1 tablespoon lime juice

1 teaspoon soy sauce

1 teaspoon chopped fresh garlic

1 teaspoon chopped fresh ginger

½ teaspoon dried ground red chile

½ cup firm tofu, cut into 1-inch cubes

1 teaspoon vegetable oil

¼ cup coarsely chopped bok choy

¼ cup coarsely chopped broccoli florets

1 small carrot, peeled and cut into thin strips

⅓ cup bean sprouts

½ cup cooked rice

1 egg (optional)

1. In a small dish, combine the lime juice, soy sauce, garlic, ginger, and red chile. Whisk until well combined. Add the tofu and marinate for at least 10 minutes and up to 2 hours. Drain the tofu, reserving the marinade.

2. In a large frying pan over high heat, warm the vegetable oil. Add the tofu and cook for 1 minute. Add the bok choy, broccoli, carrot, and bean sprouts, and cook for 2 minutes more, stirring continuously.

3. Add the cooked rice and reserved marinade to the pan. Then add the egg (if using), stirring continuously to break up the egg. Cook until the egg is scrambled, about 3 minutes.

REMIX TIPS:

→ You can replace the tofu with ¼ pound diced chicken, pork, or beef. Skip marinating the meat and season it with salt and pepper. Cook, stirring often, for 12 minutes, or until meat is cooked through. Then proceed with the rest of the recipe as written.

→ Mix in other fresh or frozen vegetables, like green beans, snap peas, onion, and baby corn cobs.

Buffalo Toaster Oven Chicken Sliders

PREP TIME: 5 minutes **COOK TIME:** 10 minutes **TOTAL TIME:** 15 minutes

These two-bite sandwiches are a fun and easy comfort food, a surefire motivator to finish studying so that you can indulge. This recipe adds a buffalo sauce, but the sliders present plenty of opportunity for customization: Add different cheeses, sauces, or spices to make them your own. For easy cleanup, line the toaster oven tray with aluminum foil before cooking. **SERVES: 1**

4 frozen pre-cooked white meat chicken nuggets

1 slice cheddar cheese, quartered

4 dinner rolls (like King's Hawaiian Rolls)

1 large lettuce leaf, cut in 4 pieces

2 tablespoons butter

½ teaspoon minced garlic

⅓ cup hot sauce

1. Put the chicken nuggets on the toaster oven tray. Top each nugget with a slice of cheese. Put the tray in the toaster oven and bake at 350°F for 10 minutes.

2. While the nuggets bake, place lettuce on the bottom half of each roll, along with any other toppings you desire (See Remix Tip below for ideas).

3. In a small microwave-safe bowl, add the butter and microwave on high for 30 seconds, or until the butter melts. Whisk in the garlic and hot sauce until the butter is incorporated into the buffalo sauce.

4. Remove the nuggets from oven and place one nugget on each prepared roll. Serve with buffalo sauce for dipping or spoon it onto the sandwiches.

REMIX TIP: Add sliced tomatoes, mayonnaise, mustard, onion, Simple Barbecue Sauce (page 167), or any of your favorite toppings.

Pasta Aglio e Olio

PREP TIME: 3 minutes **COOK TIME:** 12 minutes **TOTAL TIME:** 15 minutes

Pasta aglio e olio ("garlic and oil") is one of the simplest yet most delicious pasta dishes. The dish reportedly originated with poor Italian farmers who had nothing but the most basic ingredients to work with. This recipe uses grated Parmesan, but I encourage you to experiment with other grated hard cheeses, like Mizithra, Asiago, Pecorino, and Parmigiano-Reggiano. **SERVES: 1**

2 ounces spaghetti (see Smart Shopping Tip)

2 tablespoons extra-virgin olive oil

1 garlic clove, minced

2 tablespoons grated Parmesan cheese

1. Cook the spaghetti according to the package directions. Drain it and transfer it to a plate.

2. In a medium frying pan over medium-low heat, warm the olive oil for 2 minutes. Add the garlic and cook for 30 seconds more, or until fragrant.

3. Pour the olive oil/garlic mixture over the spaghetti and sprinkle with cheese.

REMIX TIPS:

→ Add a can of drained clams to the olive oil in step 2 and cook for 3 minutes, or until clams are heated, for clam pasta aglio e olio.

→ Add ¼ cup fresh baby spinach to the warmed olive oil and cook just until wilted, then add the garlic.

→ Add ¼ cup sliced mushrooms to the warmed olive oil and cook just until they begin to turn color, then add the garlic.

SMART SHOPPING TIP: To measure one serving of spaghetti (about 2 ounces), hold it in your hand and look at the tips. One serving should be the diameter of a US quarter.

APPLIANCE SWITCH-UP TIP: In a small microwave-safe bowl, combine the garlic and olive oil. Cover with a paper towel, and microwave on high for 1 minute. Whisk lightly and spoon over the prepared spaghetti (see Rice and Pasta in the Microwave, page 16).

Microwave Macaroni and Cheese

PREP TIME: 7 minutes **COOK TIME:** 8 minutes **TOTAL TIME:** 15 minutes

After a rough study session, what could be better than coming home to the quintessential comfort food, mac and cheese? Eat this classic version or spice it up to your liking using the add-ins below or your own imagination. **SERVES: 1**

1 cup elbow macaroni

½ cup water

⅛ teaspoon freshly ground black pepper

¼ teaspoon salt

1 tablespoon butter

1 tablespoon all-purpose flour

½ cup dairy, nut, or soy milk

⅛ teaspoon Worcestershire sauce

1 cup shredded cheddar cheese, divided (see Remix Tip)

2 tablespoons butter cracker crumbs (about 3 crackers)

1. In a deep microwave-safe bowl, combine the pasta, water, pepper, and salt, and stir. Cook on high in the microwave for 2 minutes. Stir and set aside.

2. In a small microwave-safe dish, heat the butter on high for 30 seconds, or until melted.

3. Stir the flour into butter, then whisk in the milk until smooth. Add the Worcestershire sauce and ½ cup of shredded cheese, and whisk until smooth.

4. Pour the cheese sauce over the noodles and stir until the noodles are coated. Sprinkle with cracker crumbs and microwave on medium-high for 5 minutes. Top with the remaining ½ cup of cheese.

REMIX TIP: Consider these additions: 2 strips crumbled cooked bacon; chopped scallions; ⅛ teaspoon hot sauce. Or make a cheese blend using a combination of cheddar, American, Colby, Pepper Jack, provolone, and/or mozzarella.

SMART SHOPPING: Buy block cheese and shred it yourself. The pre-shredded cheese is coated with preservatives to keep the shreds from clumping together in the bag. Shredding it yourself will yield a creamier sauce.

Chicken Parmesan

PREP TIME: 15 minutes **COOK TIME:** 15 minutes **TOTAL TIME:** 30 minutes

Chicken Parmesan is a North American dish inspired by traditional eggplant Parmesan from southern Italy. This recipe saves you from having to dredge chicken in egg and bread crumbs in your small work space; you'll achieve the same texture and flavor from a cornmeal and Parmesan cheese mixture. It comes together quickly, so keep an eye on the oven when you move to the broiling stage. **SERVES: 1**

Nonstick cooking spray

1 tablespoon grated Parmesan cheese

1 teaspoon cornmeal

¼ teaspoon dried oregano

1 boneless, skinless chicken breast

1 teaspoon extra-virgin olive oil

1 whole-wheat sandwich bun

¼ cup marinara sauce

1 slice Swiss cheese

1. Preheat the oven to 400°F and line a baking sheet with foil. Lightly spray the foil with cooking spray.

2. In a small bowl, combine the Parmesan cheese, cornmeal, and oregano. Brush the chicken with olive oil and sprinkle with the cheese mixture.

3. Put the chicken on the baking sheet and bake on the center rack for 12 minutes, or until the internal temperature reaches 165°F. Remove the chicken from the oven.

4. Turn the oven to broil and carefully move the rack from the center position to the top position (if using an oven).

5. Put the chicken on the bun and place the sandwich, open-faced, on the baking sheet. Top the chicken with marinara sauce and Swiss cheese.

6. Broil for 2 minutes, or until the cheese melts.

REMIX TIP: Change it up and make it faster by subbing in frozen pre-cooked meatballs (see package for single-serving portion) to make a meatball Parmesan sandwich.

Microwave Beef and Broccoli

PREP TIME: 15 minutes **COOK TIME:** 10 minutes **TOTAL TIME:** 25 minutes

Skip the Chinese takeout. You can make it in half of the time, for half the cost. To save even more time when you're hungry, prepare the marinade before class and then start on step 3 when you're ready to eat. **SERVES: 1**

4 teaspoons soy sauce, divided

½ teaspoon minced garlic

⅛ teaspoon grated fresh ginger

½ pound boneless beef sirloin steak, cut into thin, bite-size pieces

2 teaspoons vegetable oil

¼ cup water

2 teaspoons cornstarch

1½ cups broccoli florets

½ cup hot cooked brown or white rice (see Rice and Pasta in the Microwave, page 16)

MAKE IT EVEN FASTER:
Put the beef sirloin steak in the freezer for 1 hour before slicing; partially frozen meat is easier to slice thinly than room-temperature meat.

1. In a small mixing bowl, combine 2 teaspoons of soy sauce, the garlic, and the ginger. Whisk together until well combined.

2. Add the steak pieces to the sauce mixture and stir to coat the meat. Marinate for at least 10 minutes.

3. In a 1-quart microwave-safe dish, heat the oil in the microwave on high for 1 minute.

4. Add the beef and marinade to the oil, reduce the microwave power to medium-high, and cook for 3 minutes, or until the beef is no longer pink. Remove the meat from the liquid and set both aside.

5. In a small mixing bowl, combine the water, the remaining 2 teaspoons of soy sauce, and the cornstarch. Whisk until the cornstarch dissolves.

6. Stir the cornstarch mixture into the reserved liquid in the quart dish. Add the broccoli and stir to coat. Cover with plastic wrap and microwave on high for 5 minutes, or until the broccoli is tender and the sauce begins to thicken.

7. Uncover and add the meat back to the sauce and broccoli, stirring to coat. Microwave on high for 30 seconds to re-heat the meat. Serve over rice.

Wild Rice and Baked Salmon

PREP TIME: 10 minutes **COOK TIME:** 20 minutes **TOTAL TIME:** 30 minutes

This creamy, mushroom-y dinner is perfect before an all-night study session. Salmon is a brain food; it is chock-full of omega-3s, which are said to increase oxygen to the brain, making it easy to retain new information while holding onto information you already have. **SERVES: 1**

1 cup instant wild rice

½ tablespoon butter

¼ tablespoon extra-virgin olive oil

½ cup thinly sliced white mushrooms

¼ cup thinly sliced onion

⅛ tablespoon dried oregano

¼ teaspoon salt

⅛ teaspoon freshly ground black pepper

3 lemon slices, thinly sliced

1 salmon fillet

1 tablespoon orange juice

1 tablespoon sour cream

APPLIANCE SWITCH-UP

TIP: Try making this in the toaster oven using the same instructions but baking for 10 minutes.

1. Preheat the oven to 425°F.

2. Prepare the rice according to package directions (or see Rice and Pasta in the Microwave, page 16).

3. While the rice is cooking, in a large frying pan, heat the butter and oil over medium-high heat. Once the butter has melted, about 1 minute, add the mushrooms and onion. Cook, stirring occasionally, about 6 minutes, or until the mushrooms begin to give off their liquid and the onions are translucent. Add the oregano, salt, and pepper and stir. Remove the mushrooms and onions from the pan and set aside.

4. Fold a 12-by-12-inch piece of aluminum foil in half and then open it. Place the lemon slices along the fold, and then set the salmon fillet on top. Cover the salmon with the mushrooms and onions, then add the orange juice and sour cream.

5. Fold the foil over the salmon and crimp the edges to create a sealed pouch. Place the foil pouch on a baking sheet on the center rack of the oven and bake for 12 minutes, or until the salmon flakes. Serve with the rice.

REMIX TIP: Substitute honey, vegetable or chicken broth, or lime juice for the orange juice for a flavor variation.

Southwestern Ham and Eggs

PREP TIME: 5 minutes **COOK TIME:** 20 minutes **TOTAL TIME:** 25 minutes

Dr. Seuss knew it all along. … Ham and eggs make for great flavor.
Add potatoes and cheese for a meal you will savor.
Spread hash browns thin so they brown in a flash.
Cook them a bit longer for a crispier hash. **SERVES: 1**

- 1 tablespoon extra-virgin olive oil, divided
- ½ cup chopped cooked ham steak (see Smart Shopping Tip)
- ¼ cup chopped onion
- 1 cup frozen shredded hash browns, store-bought (or see Make It Yourself tip)
- 1 large egg
- 1 tablespoon dairy, nut, or soy milk
- ¼ teaspoon salt
- ⅛ teaspoon freshly ground black pepper
- ¼ cup shredded cheddar cheese
- 1 tablespoon salsa

1. In a medium frying pan over medium heat, warm 2 teaspoons of olive oil. Add the ham and onion, and cook until the onion is translucent, about 5 minutes. Remove from heat and transfer to a plate.

2. Drizzle the remaining 1 teaspoon of olive oil into the frying pan and warm over medium heat. Add the frozen hash browns. Cook without stirring until they begin to turn brown, about 4 minutes.

3. In a small bowl, whisk together the egg, milk, salt, and pepper and pour it into the frying pan with the hash browns. Lift the edges of the egg as it sets to allow any uncooked egg to flow under and cook. Once the egg is set, after about 4 minutes, add the ham and onion mixture. Sprinkle with cheese and cook until the cheese melts, about 3 minutes. Top with salsa.

REMIX TIPS:

→   Add 2 tablespoons frozen peas or diced green chiles to switch it up a bit.

→   Make it a meal to go by rolling the mixture into a tortilla.

MAKE IT YOURSELF TIP: To make homemade hash browns, fill a small bowl halfway with ice water. Wash and peel 1 russet potato. Using the large holes of a grater, grate the potato. Put the grated potato in the ice water and let sit for 3 minutes to remove the starch. Drain through a colander and rinse under cold water. Transfer the rinsed grated potatoes to a stack of four paper towels and gently squeeze them over the sink to remove excess water. They're now ready for this recipe.

SMART SHOPPING TIP: You can find cooked ham in the grocery store next to the other pork items like bacon or sausage. Look for "ham steak."

Roasted Vegetable Gyro

PREP TIME: 15 minutes **COOK TIME:** 15 minutes **TOTAL TIME:** 30 minutes

Tzatziki, a yogurt-cucumber sauce of Greek origin, can serve many delicious purposes. It can be a condiment for sandwiches (gyros), a sauce for meats, or a dipping appetizer all on its own. This gyro is made from tasty roasted vegetables tucked in a whole-wheat pita and topped with the creamy, tangy sauce. Make the tzatziki ahead of time and use as a dip for your favorite finger foods. **SERVES: 1**

For the tzatziki

½ cup grated cucumber

⅓ cup plain Greek yogurt

½ tablespoon extra-virgin olive oil

½ tablespoon chopped fresh dill

¼ tablespoon lemon juice

¼ teaspoon minced garlic

⅛ teaspoon salt

1. **To make the tzatziki:** Put the grated cucumber in the center of two layers of paper towels and, over a sink, lightly squeeze to remove excess moisture. Transfer the cucumber to a small serving bowl.

2. Add the yogurt, olive oil, dill, lemon juice, garlic, and salt to the cucumber, and stir until well combined. Let rest for at least 5 minutes before using.

3. **To make the gyro:** Preheat the oven to 425°F. Line an 8-by-8-inch baking pan with aluminum foil and spray lightly with cooking spray.

4. Put the carrot, sweet potato, onion, zucchini, and garlic in the baking pan.

5. In a small bowl, combine the olive oil, rosemary, brown sugar, salt, and pepper. Drizzle over the vegetables and toss to coat.

For the gyro

Nonstick cooking spray

1 large carrot, peeled and cut into 2-inch slices

1 cup diced sweet potato

1 small red onion, peeled and sliced into ½-inch slices

1 small zucchini, sliced into ¼-inch slices

1 garlic clove, minced

1 tablespoon extra-virgin olive oil

½ teaspoon dried rosemary, crushed

½ teaspoon packed brown sugar

¼ teaspoon salt

⅛ teaspoon freshly ground black pepper

1 whole-wheat pita pocket

6. Roast, uncovered, for about 15 minutes, or until the vegetables are lightly browned and tender, stirring twice during cooking.

7. Five minutes before the vegetables are to come out of the oven, place the pita bread on the oven rack to "toast."

8. Remove the pita and vegetables from the oven and fill the pita pocket with vegetables. Top with tzatziki.

REMIX TIP: The tzatziki will keep, covered, in the refrigerator for up to 4 days. It makes a great dip for raw vegetables, crackers, and more.

Apple and Sweet Potato Pork Chop

PREP TIME: 5 minutes **COOK TIME:** 45 minutes **TOTAL TIME:** 50 minutes

This might be just the recipe for a lazy winter Sunday. It may take a bit longer, but it's an all-in-one meal with a main and a side dish, so it's worth the effort. It balances the savoriness of a tender pork chop with the sweetness of apples, a classic pairing. **SERVES: 1**

½ teaspoon vegetable oil

1 (½-inch-thick) boneless pork chop

1 tablespoon brown sugar

1 tablespoon water

1 tablespoon raisins

½ tablespoon soy sauce

½ tablespoon Worcestershire sauce

1 small onion, sliced into ½-inch-thick pieces

¼ cup diced Granny Smith apple

¼ cup peeled and diced sweet potato

1. Preheat the oven to 350°F. Line an 8-by-8-inch baking dish with aluminum foil.

2. In a large frying pan over medium heat, warm the oil for 2 minutes. Add the pork chop and cook for 4 minutes on each side, or until browned.

3. While the pork chop is cooking, in a small bowl, combine the brown sugar, water, raisins, soy sauce, and Worcestershire, and mix until combined.

4. Move the browned pork chop to the baking dish and top with the onion, apple, and sweet potato. Spoon the raisin mixture over the topping.

5. Cover the dish with aluminum foil and place it on the center rack in the oven. Bake for 35 minutes, or until it reaches an internal temperature of 165°F.

REMIX TIP: Substitute another dried fruit, like cranberries, apricots, or pineapple, for the raisins.

French Bread Pizza

PREP TIME: 5 minutes **COOK TIME:** 10 minutes **TOTAL TIME:** 15 minutes

As scrumptious as pizza delivery, you can make this simple pizza in 15 minutes or less. You'll enjoy a crisp crust with just the toppings you want—what could be better for that midnight snack? **SERVES: 1**

¼ loaf French bread

2 tablespoons pizza sauce

½ teaspoon dried oregano

½ teaspoon dried basil

Additional toppings of your choice (optional): 16 pepperoni slices; ¼ cup diced, cooked chicken; sliced black olives; mushrooms; ½ cup baby spinach

¼ cup shredded mozzarella cheese

1. Preheat the oven to 400°F and line a baking sheet with aluminum foil.

2. Cut the bread in half lengthwise. You may need to thinly slice the bottom of each piece so it rests upright on the baking sheet.

3. Put the bread, cut-side up, on the baking sheet.

4. Spread 1 tablespoon of pizza sauce on each half of the bread and sprinkle with the oregano and basil. Add any additional toppings of your choice, followed by the shredded cheese.

5. Bake on the center rack for 10 minutes, or until the bread is toasted and the cheese is melted.

REMIX TIPS:

→ This is a great meal to clear out leftovers. Consider deli meats, meatloaf, and other suitable ingredients for toppings.

→ For a "thinner crust" pizza, cut the French bread in half, then halve each half again for 4 slices.

10-Minute Miso Soup

PREP TIME: 5 minutes **COOK TIME:** 5 minutes **TOTAL TIME:** 10 minutes

Typically made with fermented soybeans, salt, and rice, miso is a flavorful seasoning paste that originated in Japan. Use it to add savory flavor to this speedy, microwavable soup. This meal for one doesn't require a lot of effort, but it still has oodles of flavor and lots of plant-based protein from the edamame. Look for miso paste in the refrigerated section of your grocery store and add it at the end of the cooking process to preserve more of its heat-sensitive probiotics. This would be delicious served as a side with Microwave Beef and Broccoli (page 84). **SERVES: 1**

¼ cup frozen shelled edamame (massage the bag to help separate the beans)

¼ cup diced fresh shiitake or cremini mushrooms

1 small scallion, both white and green parts, chopped

1½ cups water

1½ tablespoons miso paste

¼ teaspoon sesame seeds (optional)

1. In a large, microwave-safe mug or bowl, stir together the edamame, mushrooms, scallion, and water. Place a paper towel on top and microwave on high for 2 minutes.

2. Carefully remove the mug from the microwave and stir.

3. Spoon the miso paste into another small bowl.

4. Pour about ¼ cup of liquid from the cooked soup into the miso and use a fork or small whisk to mix.

5. Pour the miso mixture into the soup and stir until evenly mixed.

6. Garnish with sesame seeds (if using) and serve immediately.

REMIX TIP: If you do not have mushrooms, try substituting broccoli or baby bok choy for the vegetables in this soup. Frozen (blanched and chopped) vegetables are also convenient options because you can add them to the soup without thawing.

Mediterranean Flatbread

PREP TIME: 15 minutes **TOTAL TIME:** 15 minutes

This is the perfect fried food—as in, the perfect food to make when it has been a crazy long day, your brain is fried, and you want to eat something good right now that you could practically whip up in your sleep. Keep these ingredients on hand and you will be able to make this in a snap.

SERVES: 1

½ cucumber, chopped

¼ cup pitted Kalamata olives, halved

¼ cup grape tomatoes, halved

2 teaspoons extra-virgin olive oil

1 teaspoon lemon juice

⅛ teaspoon salt

1 (6½-inch) pita bread

2 tablespoons Hummus (page 166), or store-bought

1. In a medium bowl, stir together the cucumber, olives, tomatoes, olive oil, lemon juice, and salt. Set aside for 10 minutes to marinate.

2. Place the pita on a work surface. Spread the hummus over the pita. Top with the vegetable mixture, relax, and eat.

REMIX TIP: Instead of pita bread, try crackers or toast.

Upgraded Instant Ramen

PREP TIME: 5 minutes **COOK TIME:** 5 minutes **TOTAL TIME:** 10 minutes

If you do not eat instant ramen your freshman year, it's like you never even went to college! But just because it is the quintessential student food doesn't mean you have to settle for something subpar. A soft-boiled egg and some veggies are the key to taking this dish from edible to amazing. **SERVES: 1**

2 cups water, divided

1 teaspoon white vinegar

1 large egg

1 (3-ounce) package instant ramen, any flavor

¼ cup frozen mixed vegetables

1 teaspoon soy sauce

Juice of ¼ lime

1 tablespoon sliced scallion, green parts only

1. In a microwave-safe mug, combine ½ cup of water and the vinegar, and crack the egg into it. Gently pierce the yolk with a fork so it doesn't explode while cooking. Microwave at 80 percent power for 50 to 55 seconds. Drain the water and set aside.

2. In a microwave-safe soup bowl, combine the ramen noodles, mixed vegetables, and the remaining 1½ cups of water, submerging the ramen without the water reaching all the way to the bowl's rim. Cover the noodles with a microwave-safe plate and cook for 2½ minutes, or until the noodles are soft and loose.

3. Stir in half the ramen seasoning packet (save the other half for when you want to make this again), soy sauce, and lime juice. Top with the egg and scallion.

REMIX TIP: Try adding ½ cup diced cooked chicken, thinly sliced cooked beef, or popcorn shrimp.

Zucchini Pasta Primavera

PREP TIME: 10 minutes **COOK TIME:** 10 minutes **TOTAL TIME:** 20 minutes

Pasta primavera is a classic spring dish featuring fresh vegetables and a light, creamy lemon sauce. I use zucchini noodles instead of pasta to make this dish even healthier. *Primavera* means "spring" in Italian, so this dish includes more seasonal vegetables. Feel free to use fresh, frozen, or canned vegetables for this recipe. I like to serve it with fresh basil leaves to really boost the fresh flavors of spring. **SERVES: 1**

2 tablespoons extra-virgin olive oil

1 yellow summer squash, diced

1 cup broccoli florets

½ cup frozen green peas

½ teaspoon salt

¼ teaspoon freshly ground black pepper

½ cup dairy, nut, or soy milk

½ cup shredded Parmesan cheese

1 tablespoon lemon juice

2½ cups zucchini noodles (store-bought or see Make it Yourself Tip)

2 torn basil leaves, for garnishing (optional)

1. In a large skillet over medium-low heat, warm the olive oil. When the oil shimmers, add the squash, broccoli, and peas. Season with salt and pepper to taste, and cook for 4 minutes, or until the vegetables are tender.

2. Add the milk, cheese, and lemon juice to the skillet, and stir until the cheese is melted, about 3 minutes.

3. Add the zucchini noodles and turn off the heat. Toss until the zucchini noodles are evenly coated with the sauce.

4. Taste and adjust the seasonings. Serve, sprinkled with basil (if using). Store in an airtight container in the refrigerator for up to 3 days.

REMIX TIP: Add a can of chickpeas (drained and rinsed) if you want to boost the protein.

MAKE IT YOURSELF TIP: If you have a spiralizer, you can spiralize the zucchini to make your own noodles. If you don't have a spiralizer, you can use a vegetable peeler to cut the zucchini lengthwise into long strips. Once you have peeled all the flesh off the zucchini, use a knife to cut skinny strips (the width you want your noodles). Place the "zoodles" on folded paper towels to absorb the moisture.

Microwave Risotto

PREP TIME: 5 minutes **COOK TIME:** 25 minutes **TOTAL TIME:** 30 minutes

Risotto is a creamy, delightful, traditional Italian rice dish packed with flavor, and, with this recipe, it's easy to make. This is an unusual recipe because even though the steps are simple and the ingredients list is short, it takes a little bit of time. But microwave risotto is well worth the wait. Once you have the basic recipe down, you can experiment with additional flavors. **SERVES: 1**

1 teaspoon butter

1 teaspoon extra-virgin olive oil

¼ cup uncooked arborio rice

⅔ cup chicken broth

1 teaspoon grated Parmesan cheese

½ teaspoon salt

¼ teaspoon freshly ground black pepper

1. In a microwave-safe bowl, combine the butter and oil and cook, uncovered, for 2 minutes on high.

2. Carefully remove the bowl from the microwave, stir in the rice, and microwave for 4 minutes on high. Pour in the broth and microwave for another 9 minutes. Stir the rice and microwave for another 9 minutes.

3. Fold in the Parmesan cheese, season with salt and pepper, and enjoy.

REMIX TIP: You can add more flavors by incorporating other seasonings, such as garlic powder. Just ¼ teaspoon can change the whole dish. You might also try 1 tablespoon fresh chopped parsley, 1 tablespoon fresh chopped chives, or even 1 cup sautéed mushrooms.

Quick Shrimp Scampi

PREP TIME: 5 minutes **COOK TIME:** 10 minutes **TOTAL TIME:** 15 minutes

"Scampi" actually refers small lobster-like creatures, but over the years it has come to represent this particular way to prepare shrimp: sautéed with butter, garlic, and lemon. The dish, though it sounds (and tastes) impressive, is incredibly easy to make. The key is to keep an eye on the shrimp as they cook. As soon as they turn pink, remove them from the heat. It's quick, so have the pasta ready. **SERVES: 1**

½ cup pasta

1 tablespoon butter

¼ pound shrimp, peeled and deveined (see Smart Shopping Tip)

1 scallion, finely sliced, both white and light green parts

½ teaspoon minced garlic

½ teaspoon chopped fresh parsley

⅛ teaspoon freshly ground black pepper

½ tablespoon lemon juice or white wine

SMART SHOPPING TIP:
You can buy frozen shrimp. Unlike chicken, frozen shrimp doesn't have to defrost; just add them directly to the pan, and add 2 minutes more to the cooking time. You can also buy pre-cooked shrimp. Add them to the pan and just cook until the shrimp are heated through.

1. Cook the pasta according to package instructions, or see Rice and Pasta in the Microwave (page 16).

2. While the pasta is cooking, melt the butter in a medium skillet over medium heat.

3. Add the shrimp, scallion, garlic, parsley, and pepper. Cook the shrimp for 3 minutes, or just until they turn pink, stirring continuously.

4. Remove from the heat and stir in the lemon juice.

5. Serve over the pasta.

REMIX TIPS:

→ Add ¼ teaspoon red pepper flakes for a spicy shrimp scampi.

→ For more flavorful noodles, sprinkle them with 1 tablespoon chopped parsley or 1 tablespoon grated Parmesan cheese before topping with the shrimp and sauce.

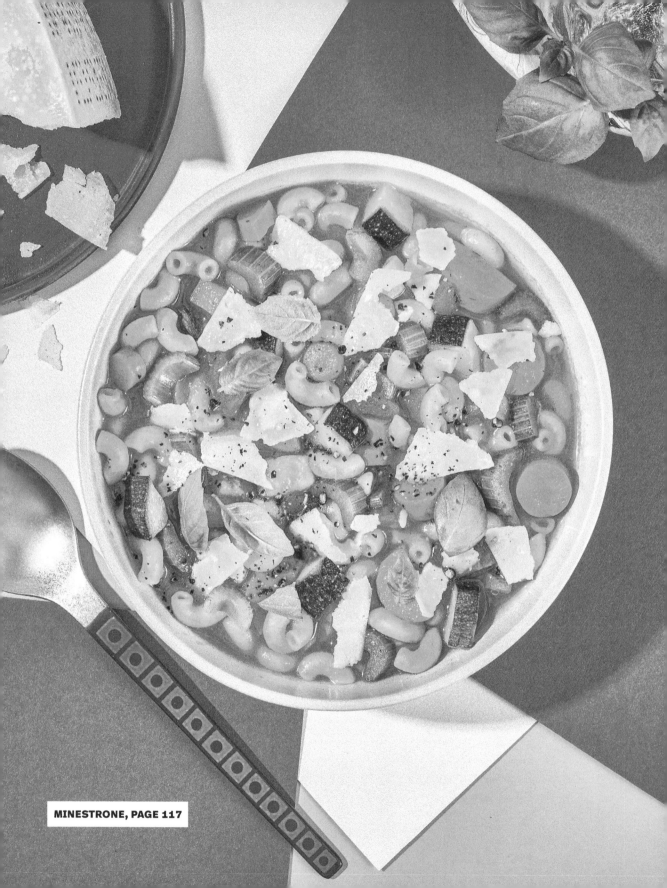

MINESTRONE, PAGE 117

7

Meals with Friends

Microwave Chili

PREP TIME: 10 minutes **COOK TIME:** 20 minutes **TOTAL TIME:** 30 minutes

Everyone needs a homemade chili recipe; it's delicious, hearty, and comforting, perfect to share with your friends for a Sunday night dinner. Make this and share or enjoy it as leftovers (I think it tastes even better the next day!). **SERVES: 6**

1 pound ground beef

1 medium yellow onion, chopped

1 garlic clove, chopped

1 (14.5-ounce) can diced tomatoes

1 (15-ounce) can kidney beans, drained

1 (8-ounce) can tomato sauce

1 (4-ounce) can diced green chiles

2 teaspoons chili powder

½ teaspoon salt

¼ teaspoon ground cumin

¼ teaspoon unsweetened cocoa

1 tablespoon strong coffee or espresso

Toppings of your choice (optional): grated cheddar cheese, sour cream, and/or chopped onion

1. In a 2-quart microwave-safe dish, combine the ground beef, onion, and garlic, and microwave on high for 5 minutes, or until the ground beef is no longer pink. Drain and break the ground beef into small chunks using a large spoon.

2. Add the tomatoes, beans, tomato sauce, chiles, chili powder, salt, cumin, cocoa, and coffee to the ground beef, and stir to combine. Cover and microwave on medium-high for 10 minutes.

3. Uncover and microwave for 5 more minutes on medium-high. Serve hot, garnished with toppings (if using).

REMIX TIPS:

→ Leave out the ground beef for vegetarian chili or replace it with a lean ground turkey for a lighter version.

→ Replace half of the ground beef with mild or hot Italian sausage.

→ Substitute canned chopped jalapeños for the green chiles.

Microwave Salisbury Steak

PREP TIME: 10 minutes **COOK TIME:** 15 minutes **TOTAL TIME:** 25 minutes

Salisbury steak is like a mash-up of meatloaf and hamburger. I like this comfort food because it offers so many options. There is the classic Salisbury steak, which pairs incredibly well with mashed potatoes. You can make Salisbury steak subs, messy but worth it. Last, but definitely not least, try Salisbury meatballs, which are a great appetizer, snack, or spaghetti topper. **SERVES: 6**

1½ pounds lean ground beef

1 (10¼-ounce) can condensed cream of mushroom soup, divided

1 (4-ounce) can sliced mushrooms, divided

½ cup bread crumbs

1 cup dairy, nut, or soy milk, divided

1 egg, slightly beaten

¼ cup minced onion

⅛ teaspoon freshly ground black pepper

2 teaspoons dried parsley flakes

1. In a large mixing bowl, combine the ground beef, ⅓ cup of condensed soup, half of the mushrooms, the bread crumbs, ½ cup of milk, the egg, onion, and pepper. Use your hands to mix the ingredients until well combined and then shape them into six 1-inch-thick patties.

2. Place the patties on a large microwave-safe plate and cover with wax paper. Microwave on high for 5 minutes. Turn the patties over and microwave on high for 5 minutes more, or until the patties are no longer pink. Drain.

3. While the patties are cooking, in a small bowl, combine the remaining soup, mushrooms, and milk with the parsley. Mix until well combined.

4. Pour the mixture over the beef patties and microwave on high for 5 minutes, or until heated through.

REMIX TIPS:

→ Slice sub rolls in half lengthwise, add patties, top with gravy, and sprinkle with shredded Swiss cheese for a Salisbury steak sub.

→ Form the meat mixture into 1½-inch meatballs, place on a microwave-safe baking dish, and microwave on medium for 7 minutes. Add gravy and microwave on medium for 8 minutes more, or until the meatballs are firm.

Lasagna

PREP TIME: 13 minutes **COOK TIME:** 32 minutes **TOTAL TIME:** 45 minutes

Impress your roommates with this easy lasagna. Serve it with a side salad and a loaf of Italian bread for a complete and elegant meal. You can assemble this ahead of time: Just freeze and then thaw before baking and eating. Feel free to add your own twist with different cheeses.

SERVES: 4

Nonstick cooking spray

1 pound ground beef

1 small onion, chopped

½ cup small-curd cottage cheese

½ cup grated mozzarella cheese

1 egg, beaten

½ teaspoon salt

¼ teaspoon garlic powder

2½ cups marinara sauce, divided

4 lasagna noodles, cooked and cut in half widthwise

¼ cup shredded cheddar cheese

MAKE IT EVEN FASTER:
Use pre-cooked lasagna noodles for even faster preparation.

1. Preheat the oven to 425°F and spray an 8-by-8-inch baking dish with cooking spray.

2. In a large frying pan over medium heat, cook the ground beef and onion for 7 minutes, or until the ground beef is no longer pink and the onion is translucent.

3. While the ground beef is cooking, in a medium bowl, combine the cottage cheese, mozzarella, egg, salt, and garlic powder, and stir.

4. Drain the ground beef and add 2 cups of marinara sauce. Stir to combine.

5. Spread out half of the ground beef mixture in the bottom of the baking dish. Add 4 of the lasagna noodle halves. Top with half of the cottage cheese mixture. Repeat.

6. Top with the remaining ½ cup of marinara and the shredded cheddar cheese.

7. Place on the center rack of the preheated oven and bake for 25 minutes.

REMIX TIP: Eliminate the meat altogether and make a veggie lasagna by sautéing 1 chopped bell pepper, 1 small chopped zucchini, and 1 cup baby spinach along with the onion in 1 tablespoon olive oil for 7 minutes, or until the vegetables are tender.

Thai Peanut Noodles

PREP TIME: 15 minutes **COOK TIME:** 5 minutes **TOTAL TIME:** 20 minutes

Thai peanut noodles have a perfect balance of the four "S"s: salty, sweet, spicy, and savory. If you're buying the peanut sauce and are eating vegetarian, read the label, because sometimes these sauces contain fish sauce. To be completely safe, make your own tangy peanut sauce with the recipe provided in the Make It Yourself Tip. **SERVES: 2**

4 ounces thin rice noodles

4 cups boiling water

2 tablespoons vegetable oil

2 eggs, whisked

2 scallions, thinly sliced

1 carrot, shredded

½ cup Thai peanut sauce

1. In a heatproof dish, cover the rice noodles with the boiling water. Allow them to soften for 10 minutes, then drain in a colander.

2. Heat a large skillet over medium heat until hot, then add the oil and heat for 30 seconds more. Pour the whisked eggs into the skillet. Cook undisturbed for 1 to 2 minutes, until the eggs are set. Carefully flip the egg pancake over and cook for 30 seconds on the other side. Slide the cooked eggs onto a cutting board.

3. Place the scallions and carrot in the skillet and sauté for 30 seconds. Add the drained noodles to the pan and cook for 1 minute. Pour in the peanut sauce and cook until just heated through, about 1 minute more.

4. Slice the egg into long, thin strips and add to the noodles just before serving.

MAKE IT YOURSELF TIP: To make Thai peanut sauce: In a small jar, combine ¼ cup creamy peanut butter, 2 tablespoons soy sauce, 1 tablespoon honey or brown sugar, 2 tablespoons lime juice, 1 teaspoon minced ginger, ¼ teaspoon red pepper flakes, and 1 teaspoon minced garlic. Cover the jar tightly with a lid and shake vigorously until combined.

Microwave Spaghetti and Meatballs

PREP TIME: 15 minutes **COOK TIME:** 25 minutes **TOTAL TIME:** 40 minutes

Classic spaghetti and meatballs is a great dish to have in your arsenal, and it doesn't need to be a big production. In fact, it can be made in the microwave—including the pasta. It's important to let the dish rest before eating. Serve with a side salad and dinner rolls for a wholesome meal.

SERVES: 4 TO 6

½ pound ground beef

¼ pound ground pork

½ small onion, finely minced

½ cup dairy, nut, or soy milk

½ egg, lightly beaten

½ cup bread crumbs

½ teaspoon salt

⅛ teaspoon freshly ground black pepper

1 (28-ounce) jar marinara sauce

2 cups water

8 ounces spaghetti

1 garlic clove, minced

½ cup grated cheddar cheese

1. In a large mixing bowl, combine the beef, pork, onion, milk, egg, bread crumbs, salt, and pepper with your hands until well incorporated. Shape the mixture into 1½-inch meatballs.

2. In a 3-quart microwave-safe dish, arrange the meatballs in a single layer and cook on medium for 4 minutes.

3. Add the marinara sauce, water, spaghetti, and garlic. Stir, cover, and microwave on high for 5 minutes. Stir, cover, and microwave for 10 minutes more. Stir.

4. Add the cheese. Cover and microwave on high for 5 minutes, or until the noodles are tender. Remove from the microwave and stir. Allow the dish to rest for 5 minutes before serving.

REMIX TIP: For a chunkier sauce, add 1 (28-ounce) can diced tomatoes with their liquid in place of water. If the pasta is still exposed, add just enough water to cover it completely.

MAKE IT EVEN FASTER TIP: You can save prep time by purchasing frozen meatballs and preparing them according to package directions, or use your leftover Microwave Salisbury Steak (page 101) meatballs.

Microwave Peach Chicken

PREP TIME: 10 minutes **COOK TIME:** 20 minutes **TOTAL TIME:** 30 minutes

This microwave peach chicken offers a sweet, tangy, and refreshing flavor. Diced peaches boost the flavor and add a pop of color and texture. Make sure you use jam or preserves rather than jelly for the best results. Whereas jelly is made with strained fruit, jam is made from mashed fruit and preserves actually retain some fruit pieces, so both jam and preserves have a more intense fruitiness than jelly. **SERVES: 4**

1 cup peach jam

½ cup French
  salad dressing

1 envelope onion
  soup mix

½ cup diced peaches,
  canned or fresh
  and peeled

¼ cup mayonnaise

8 skin-on
  chicken drumsticks

1. In an 8-by-8-inch microwave-safe dish, combine the jam, dressing, onion soup mix, peaches, and mayonnaise, and stir until well combined.

2. Add the chicken to the dish and turn once to coat, placing the thicker ends toward the outside of the dish.

3. Cover with plastic wrap and use a fork to poke holes in the center to allow venting. Microwave on high for 8 minutes.

4. Turn the chicken over, re-cover the dish, and cook for 12 minutes, or until the chicken is opaque. The chicken may still be slightly rare near the bone, but it will keep cooking in the next step.

5. Let the chicken rest for 5 minutes. Use a meat thermometer to ensure that the internal temperature has reached 165°F.

REMIX TIPS:

→ Substitute ½ cup sliced strawberries for the diced peaches.

→ Add 1 small jalapeño, seeded and sliced.

Curry Quesadillas

PREP TIME: 10 minutes **COOK TIME:** 15 minutes **TOTAL TIME:** 25 minutes

Quesadillas make very versatile vessels for various vibrant fillings. This recipe uses curry to change up the flavor profile. But the other fillings are limited only by your imagination. **SERVES: 4**

3 teaspoons vegetable oil, divided

¼ cup diced onion

1 garlic clove, minced

2 teaspoons curry powder

¼ teaspoon red pepper flakes

1 (15.5-ounce) can vegetarian refried beans

1 large globe or beefsteak tomato, diced

8 (8-inch) flour tortillas

1. In a large frying pan over medium heat, warm 1 teaspoon of vegetable oil for 2 minutes. Add the onion and sauté for 3 minutes, or until translucent. Stir in the garlic.

2. Once the garlic is fragrant, about 30 seconds, stir in the curry powder and red pepper flakes. Cook, stirring continuously, for 1 minute.

3. Add the beans and tomato, along with any juices released from dicing it, and cook for 3 minutes.

4. Divide the bean mixture evenly among 4 tortillas, leaving ½ inch of tortilla uncovered at the edges.

5. Add ½ teaspoon of oil to a large frying pan and warm over medium heat for 1 minute. Gently place the tortilla with the beans into the pan, and lay a second tortilla on top.

6. Cook for 2 minutes and gently turn the tortilla over in the pan. Cook 2 minutes more, or until the tortilla is golden.

7. Repeat with remaining oil and tortillas.

REMIX TIPS:

→ Try adding ½ cup finely diced red or green apple and ½ cup chopped baby spinach along with the bean mixture.

→ Add 1 cup chopped or shredded rotisserie chicken along with the bean mixture for a curry chicken quesadilla.

Chicken Noodle Soup

PREP TIME: 10 minutes **COOK TIME:** 15 minutes **TOTAL TIME:** 25 minutes

Nurture yourself, and your dorm-mates, with this must-have recipe straight from the kitchen of my grandmother Charlotte the Great. It's a basic chicken noodle soup recipe, but who doesn't love that? Use leftover or store-bought rotisserie chicken to keep the prep time down. Grandma's version includes the thickened cream in the Remix Tip.

SERVES: 4

- 2 teaspoons extra-virgin olive oil
- 1 small onion, chopped
- 2 garlic cloves, minced
- 2 small celery stalks, chopped
- 1 medium carrot, peeled and chopped
- ½ teaspoon salt
- ¾ teaspoon freshly ground black pepper
- 4 cups chicken broth
- 4 cups water
- 1½ teaspoons dried oregano
- 1⅓ cups shredded cooked chicken
- 2 cups cooked egg noodles
- ¼ cup chopped fresh parsley or chives, for garnish

1. In a large pot over medium heat, combine the olive oil, onion, garlic, celery, and carrot. Sauté for 4 minutes, or until the celery and carrot are tender and the onion is translucent. Season with salt and pepper.

2. Add the chicken broth, water, and oregano, and bring to a full boil.

3. Add the chicken and return the soup to a boil. Reduce the heat to medium-low and cook for 5 minutes to fuse the flavors.

4. Add the cooked noodles and return to a simmer. Serve garnished with chopped fresh parsley or chives. This soup keeps in an airtight container in the refrigerator for up to 3 days.

REMIX TIPS:

→ For a creamy chicken noodle soup, add 2 to 4 tablespoons of heavy cream, half-and-half, or whole milk.

→ For a thickened creamy chicken noodle soup, make a slurry by whisking 1 tablespoon cornstarch with 2 tablespoons heavy cream. Stir into the soup as it boils, until slightly thickened.

→ Swap the noodles for rice or a diced sweet potato.

Ground Beef Tacos

PREP TIME: 5 minutes **COOK TIME:** 10 minutes **TOTAL TIME:** 15 minutes

This Mexican street food has become ubiquitous around the world, and it's no wonder why: Tacos are so tasty and easy to make. Here, I love the flavor combination of beans, salsa, and ground beef—and this mixture helps keep the ground beef inside the taco shell. **SERVES: 4**

1 pound ground beef

1 small onion, chopped

¼ teaspoon salt

1 (1-ounce) package taco seasoning

1 cup refried beans

¾ cup salsa

8 taco shells or warmed corn tortillas

1 cup shredded lettuce

1 cup shredded cheddar cheese

1. Heat a large frying pan over medium heat for 2 minutes. Add the ground beef and onion. Cook for 5 minutes, stirring often to break up the ground beef, until the onion is translucent. Drain the excess liquid. Add the salt and taco seasoning and stir.

2. Stir in the refried beans and salsa and cook 2 minutes, or until heated through.

3. Divide the meat mixture among the taco shells and top each with lettuce, cheese, and any other favorite toppings.

REMIX TIPS:

→ To make this vegan, omit the cheese (or replace with a nondairy version) and ground beef. You can substitute crumbled tofu for the ground beef.

→ Make a taco bar by filling bowls with your favorite taco toppings–sour cream, black olives, green chiles, jalapeños, salsa, varieties of shredded cheese–and let each guest create their own.

Shakshuka

PREP TIME: 5 minutes **COOK TIME:** 15 minutes **TOTAL TIME:** 20 minutes

This one-pan vegetarian meal is perfect for a savory breakfast or a filling dinner. For added protein, consider adding cooked white beans to the pan just before adding the eggs, and top with crumbled feta cheese.

SERVES: 2 to 4

3 tablespoons
  extra-virgin olive oil

4 garlic cloves, smashed

1 onion, halved and
  thinly sliced

3 bell peppers, red,
  yellow, and orange,
  cored and thinly sliced

1 (15-ounce) can
  fire-roasted diced
  tomatoes, drained

Sea salt

Freshly ground
  black pepper

4 eggs

¼ cup roughly chopped
  fresh parsley,
  for garnish

1. In a large skillet, heat the olive oil over medium heat. Cook the garlic and onion for 5 minutes, until they begin to soften.

2. Add the bell peppers and cook for another 5 minutes.

3. Add the tomatoes and bring the mixture a simmer. Season with salt and pepper.

4. Using a large spoon, make four indentations in the vegetable mixture, and crack an egg into each one. Cook, uncovered, until the whites are set and the egg yolks are still runny, about 5 minutes. Garnish with fresh parsley.

REMIX TIP: Shakshuka is traditionally spiced with ground cumin, smoked paprika, and cayenne pepper. If you have these spices in your pantry, add ¼ teaspoon of each to your shakshuka before adding the eggs.

Herb-Crusted Salmon

PREP TIME: 10 minutes **COOK TIME:** 10 minutes **TOTAL TIME:** 20 minutes

Salmon is among the healthiest fish and makes one of the best brain foods. So amp up the brain power for you and all of your study partners with this delicious take on salmon. The delicate herb crust is sure to impress even the most discerning college foodie. Pair the salmon with sautéed greens to add some color and even more nutrients to the plate.

SERVES: 4

Nonstick cooking spray

1 pound salmon fillets

1 teaspoon extra-virgin olive oil

¼ teaspoon salt

¼ teaspoon freshly ground black pepper

1 cup bread crumbs

1 tablespoon dried parsley

1 tablespoon dried tarragon

2 eggs, beaten

1 lemon, cut into 4 wedges

1. Preheat the oven to 425°F. Line a baking sheet with aluminum foil and lightly spray with cooking spray.

2. Divide the salmon into 4 equal pieces. Drizzle with the olive oil and season with salt and pepper.

3. In a medium bowl, combine the bread crumbs, parsley, and tarragon, and mix to combine.

4. Dip the salmon in the beaten eggs, and then dredge it in the bread-crumb mixture, coating all sides. Put the coated salmon fillets on the foil-lined baking sheet.

5. Stir any remaining egg into the leftover bread crumbs, and top each piece of salmon with some of the bread crumb mixture.

6. Place on the center rack of the oven and bake for 5 minutes, or until just a little bit of pink is left in the middle of the salmon.

7. Broil the salmon for 2 minutes, keeping an eye on the breading; you want it golden. Serve the salmon with lemon wedges.

REMIX TIP: Replace the bread crumbs with 1 cup crushed butter crackers for a buttery taste.

Red Beans and Rice

PREP TIME: 5 minutes **COOK TIME:** 20 minutes **TOTAL TIME:** 25 minutes

Red beans and rice is a dish I learned to love during my time in Miami. It's perfect for college because it is inexpensive, super easy, and offers protein for brain fuel, and it is versatile in that it can be a main or a side dish.

SERVES: 4

2 cups rice

1 tablespoon extra-virgin olive oil

1 small onion, coarsely chopped

1 medium green bell pepper, chopped

2 garlic cloves, crushed (see Make it Yourself Tip)

1 large tomato, chopped

1 (15-ounce) can kidney beans, drained and rinsed

1 cup tomato sauce

¼ teaspoon salt

¼ teaspoon ground cumin

¼ teaspoon hot sauce (optional)

⅓ cup water

1. Prepare the rice according to the package instructions, or see Rice and Pasta in the Microwave (page 16).

2. While the rice is cooking, in a large frying pan, warm the oil over medium-high heat for 2 minutes. Add the onion, green pepper, and garlic, and cook for 5 minutes, stirring occasionally, until the onions are translucent.

3. Add the tomato, kidney beans, tomato sauce, salt, cumin, hot sauce (if using), cooked rice, and water. Stir to combine. Reduce the heat to medium and simmer uncovered for 10 minutes.

REMIX TIP: In step 2, add 1 pound cooked ground beef, 1 pound shredded cooked chicken or pork, 1 pound sliced kielbasa, or a package of firm tofu, crumbled.

MAKE IT YOURSELF TIP: To crush garlic, peel the garlic clove and place it on a cutting board. Place your chef's knife blade on top of the clove of garlic with the sharp edge facing away from you. Use the heel of your hand (keeping fingers curled and away from the knife's edge) and press until the garlic collapses, or is "crushed."

Spaghetti Squash with Garlic Tomato Sauce

PREP TIME: 10 minutes **COOK TIME:** 45 minutes **TOTAL TIME:** 55 minutes

Want to feel like you're carb-loading when you're not? This nutritious take on a spaghetti dinner uses spaghetti squash—a high-fiber, nutrient-dense, antioxidant-rich vegetable—as "noodles" rather than pasta. The color, flavor, and textures make this recipe worth a little extra time. **SERVES: 4**

1 large spaghetti squash, cut in half lengthwise

1 tablespoon extra-virgin olive oil

2 garlic cloves, crushed (see Red Beans and Rice, Make It Yourself Tip, page 111)

1 small onion, diced

5 Roma tomatoes, sliced

¼ cup balsamic vinegar

½ teaspoon salt

¼ teaspoon freshly ground black pepper

1 (28-ounce jar) marinara sauce

½ cup grated Parmesan cheese

5 fresh basil leaves, cut into thin strips

1. Preheat the oven to 350°F.

2. Wrap each squash half in foil and place them on a baking sheet. Bake in the oven for 45 minutes, or until tender.

3. While the spaghetti squash is baking, in a large frying pan, warm the olive oil over medium heat for 2 minutes. Add the garlic, onions, and tomatoes, and cook, stirring, for 20 minutes. Add the vinegar, salt, and pepper. Stir in the marinara sauce, reduce the heat to medium-low, and simmer until ready to serve.

4. Carefully remove the spaghetti squash from the foil. Scoop out and discard the stringy fibers and seeds. With a large spoon, scoop the squash's flesh into a bowl; using 2 forks, pull apart the flesh into spaghetti-like strands.

5. Divide the spaghetti squash among plates, top with sauce, and sprinkle with cheese and basil.

REMIX TIPS:

→ Sauté 8 ounces mushrooms with the garlic and onions for an earthy taste.

→ Try garnishing with black olives.

Mustard and Maple Glazed Chicken

PREP TIME: 5 minutes **COOK TIME:** 40 minutes **TOTAL TIME:** 45 minutes

I love this recipe for its unique sweet tanginess. Your entire hall will be thanking you, because the aromas it gives off are exceptional. It has a longer cooking time but very little preparation, which seems like a great trade-off, especially when you're entertaining. **SERVES: 4**

Nonstick cooking spray

4 boneless, skinless chicken breasts (or any cut you like)

½ teaspoon salt

½ teaspoon freshly ground black pepper

½ cup Dijon mustard

¼ cup maple syrup

1 tablespoon apple cider vinegar

1 tablespoon fresh thyme

1. Preheat the oven to 450°F. Lightly spray an 8-by-8-inch baking dish with cooking spray.

2. Put the chicken in the baking dish and sprinkle with salt and pepper.

3. In a small mixing bowl, combine the mustard, maple syrup, and vinegar, and pour over the chicken.

4. Put the chicken on the center rack of the oven and bake for 40 minutes, or until the internal temperature reaches 165°F. Halfway through the bake time, spoon some of the sauce from the bottom of the pan over the chicken.

5. Remove from the oven and sprinkle with fresh thyme before serving.

REMIX TIPS:

→ If you indulge and buy chicken with the skin on for this recipe, it will be more flavorful.

→ Use 12 chicken wings and make it wing night.

Meatloaf in a Mug

PREP TIME: 15 minutes **COOK TIME:** 12 minutes **TOTAL TIME:** 27 minutes

Bring your study partner a hot, steaming mug of . . . meatloaf? Yes! These meatloaves in a mug are as portable as they are delicious. Plus, they contain all of the protein you need to study long into the night, if need be. Be sure to use extra-lean ground beef so your mug isn't filled with grease.

SERVES: 4

For the meatloaf

1 pound extra-lean ground beef (see Smart Shopping Tip below)

½ cup bread crumbs

⅛ cup grated Parmesan cheese

¼ cup finely chopped scallions

¼ cup ketchup

1 large egg

½ teaspoon minced garlic

1 teaspoon steak seasoning (optional)

½ teaspoon salt

¼ teaspoon freshly ground black pepper

1. **To make the meatloaf:** In a large bowl, combine the ground beef, bread crumbs, Parmesan cheese, scallions, ketchup, egg, garlic, steak seasoning (if using), salt, and pepper. Mix with your hands until well combined. Divide the mixture evenly into four portions and shape each into a ball.

2. Place each meatloaf ball in an 8-ounce microwave-safe mug. Place a piece of wax paper in the microwave to catch any juices and arrange the mugs in a square on top of the wax paper. Cover the mugs with one large sheet of wax paper.

3. Microwave for 11 minutes on medium-high. Using a knife and fork, cut into the center of the meatloaf; if it is still pink, cook in intervals of 30 seconds until no longer pink.

For the ooey-gooey sauce

2½ teaspoons packed brown sugar

⅓ cup ketchup

½ tablespoon dry mustard

½ teaspoon Worcestershire sauce

4. **To make the sauce:** While the meatloaves are cooking, in a small bowl, combine the sugar, ketchup, mustard, and Worcestershire sauce, and stir until the brown sugar dissolves.

5. Spoon the sauce over the top of each meatloaf mug, cover with wax paper, and let rest for 2 minutes before serving.

REMIX TIP: Top with warm mashed potatoes for a meal in a mug.

SMART SHOPPING TIP: When choosing ground beef, keep in mind that extra-lean ground beef has no more than 10 percent fat, lean ground beef has no more than 17 percent fat, medium ground beef has 20 percent fat, and regular ground beef has 30 percent fat.

Mediterranean-Inspired Chicken Rice Bowl

PREP TIME: 15 minutes **COOK TIME:** 15 minutes **TOTAL TIME:** 30 minutes

Rice bowls have so much going for them. They are packed with nutrients, colorful, and completely customizable to your tastes and moods. I use brown rice here because it is less processed than white rice, so it retains its antioxidants, vitamins, and minerals. But feel free to branch out and experiment. **SERVES: 4**

1 cup instant brown rice

1 cup chopped cooked chicken breast

1 cup chopped cucumbers

1 cup halved cherry tomatoes

1 cup sliced olives

1 cup cooked chickpeas

1 cup crumbled feta cheese

½ cup lemon juice

4 teaspoons fresh mint leaves, chopped, for garnishing

1. Cook the rice according to package instructions.

2. In a large bowl, combine the rice, chicken, cucumbers, tomatoes, olives, and chickpeas. Toss lightly to combine.

3. Sprinkle the feta cheese over the top and pour on the lemon juice to taste. Garnish with the mint and serve.

REMIX TIP: Make this vegetarian by replacing the chicken with tempeh. Use half of an 8-ounce block of tempeh and cut it into ½-inch-thick strips.

MAKE IT YOURSELF TIP: To cook raw chicken in the microwave, place 1 (3-ounce) chicken breast on a microwave-safe plate with the thickest part toward the outside of the plate. Cover with plastic wrap and poke a ¼-inch slit in the center of the plastic with a knife. Microwave on medium for 12 minutes, or until juice is clear and the chicken is no longer pink. Let the chicken rest for 5 minutes to finish cooking.

Minestrone

PREP TIME: 10 minutes **COOK TIME:** 30 minutes **TOTAL TIME:** 40 minutes

Minestrone is an Italian alternative to chicken soup when you're a bit under the weather. This recipe makes four servings, so you can share with some friends, keep some leftovers for the next day, or freeze them for the next time you feel the need for some warm and comforting soup.

SERVES: 4

2 tablespoons
 extra-virgin olive oil

½ small onion, diced

2 garlic cloves, minced

1 medium carrot, diced

1 medium celery
 stalk, diced

1 small zucchini, diced

½ (14.5-ounce) can
 diced tomatoes

3 cups vegetable broth

½ cup elbow macaroni

2 teaspoons
 Italian seasoning

½ teaspoon salt

¼ teaspoon freshly
 ground black pepper

10 fresh basil
 leaves (optional)

Shaved Parmesan
 (optional)

1. In a large saucepan, warm the oil over medium-high heat. Add the onion, garlic, carrot, celery, and zucchini, and stir well.

2. Add the diced tomatoes, broth, macaroni, Italian seasoning, salt, and pepper. Stir to combine thoroughly.

3. Bring to a boil, then simmer for 20 minutes. Taste to check that the macaroni and vegetables are fully cooked, then serve. Garnish with basil leaves and Parmesan (if using).

REMIX TIP: If you're not vegan, try replacing the elbow macaroni with cheese tortellini for a yummy twist with added protein.

Date-Night Steak and Mashed Potatoes

PREP TIME: 10 minutes **COOK TIME:** 25 minutes **TOTAL TIME:** 35 minutes

Perfectly searing a steak is not a requirement to get your degree, but it should be. Most first-timers overcook the steak, which then ends up chewy, bland, and a woeful shade of gray. The secret is to get the pan sizzling hot before adding the steaks to it. This creates what is known as the Maillard reaction, where the sugars and amino acids in the meat start to brown, giving the steak a nice crust and its irresistible savory flavor.

SERVES: 2

- 5 or 6 Yukon Gold or red potatoes (about 1 pound), peeled and quartered
- ¼ cup dairy, nut, or soy milk
- 2 teaspoons garlic powder, divided
- 2 tablespoons unsalted butter
- Salt
- Freshly ground black pepper
- 2 (8-ounce) sirloin steaks (see Smart Shopping Tip)
- 1 tablespoon vegetable oil

1. Put the potatoes in a medium saucepan, cover them with water, and bring to a boil over high heat. Reduce the heat to medium and cook the potatoes for 15 minutes, or until tender when pierced with a fork. Drain the potatoes and return them to the pot.

2. Using a potato masher or a large fork, lightly mash the potatoes. Add the milk, 1½ teaspoons of garlic powder, and the butter, mashing and mixing to combine. Season with salt and pepper to taste. Cover to keep warm and set aside.

3. Heat a skillet over medium-high heat.

4. Pat the steaks dry with a paper towel, and season both sides with salt and pepper to taste along with the remaining ½ teaspoon of garlic powder.

5. Add the vegetable oil to the skillet. If the skillet is hot enough, the oil should sizzle a little. If it doesn't sizzle, it's a sign the skillet isn't hot enough. Wait 30 seconds to 1 minute, watching the oil until its surface starts to shimmer, then add the steaks. Cook the steaks without

moving them for 4 to 5 minutes. Using a pair of tongs or a spatula, flip the steaks and cook for 2 to 3 minutes more, until the edges turn brown. To test for doneness, press the meat with your tongs—for a medium steak, it should be as tender as pressing your finger to your chin. Transfer the steaks to a cutting board to rest for a few minutes.

6. Place each steak on a plate and serve with mashed potatoes.

REMIX TIP: Herbed butter requires a little prep time (and an hour in the refrigerator), but it is well worth the effort and enhances both the steaks and mashed potatoes.

In a small bowl, mix ¼ cup softened butter, ¾ teaspoon lemon juice, ¼ teaspoon salt, ⅛ teaspoon minced garlic, ¾ tablespoon dried parsley, 2 teaspoons dried oregano, 2 teaspoons dried rosemary, and ⅛ teaspoon freshly ground black pepper until combined, then press the herbed butter into silicone molds. Alternatively, spray a nonstick tablespoon-size measuring spoon with nonstick cooking spray and press the butter mixture into the scoop, tapping the butter out onto plastic wrap. Cover with plastic wrap and refrigerate for 1 hour.

SMART SHOPPING TIP: Look for steaks with good red color. The steak should be firm but not hard, moist but not wet.

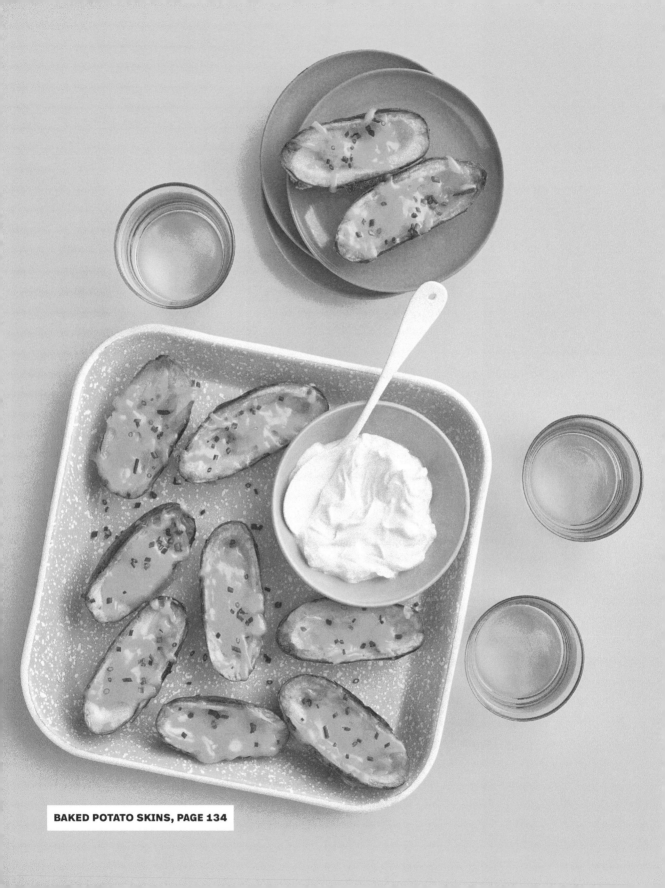

BAKED POTATO SKINS, PAGE 134

Tailgating and Party Food

Baked Chicken Wings

PREP TIME: 5 minutes **COOK TIME:** 45 minutes **TOTAL TIME:** 50 minutes

What's more of a crowd-pleaser than chicken wings? So popular! So portable! So palatable! You can bake the wings so they are less greasy than the fried ones you order in bars. They taste delicious right out of the oven, or you can toss them with or dip them in your favorite sauce. Check out the Remix Tips below for some options. **SERVES: 6 TO 8**

2 tablespoons extra-virgin olive oil

1 tablespoon salt

½ teaspoon freshly ground black pepper

5 pounds chicken wings (I buy the drumettes)

1. Preheat the oven to 400°F.

2. Set a wire rack inside each of 2 large, rimmed baking sheets. You can also place the wings directly on a foil-covered baking sheet with a catch pan underneath because they will drip.

3. In a large bowl, mix the olive oil, salt, and pepper. Add the wings and toss to coat. Divide the wings between the prepared racks and spread them out in a single layer, or arrange them in a single layer on the foil-covered baking sheet.

4. Bake the wings until cooked through and the skin is crispy, 45 to 50 minutes.

5. Remove from the oven and eat them plain, tossed in your favorite sauce, or with dipping sauces.

REMIX TIPS:

→ To go in a different flavor direction, try adding ¼ cup grated Parmesan cheese to the olive oil, salt, and pepper.

→ You can make sauces easily by heating fruit preserves in the microwave in 30-second intervals. Then brush them on the chicken wings or toss the wings in a bowl with the warm preserves. Try 1 cup blackberry preserves with 1 tablespoon adobo sauce, or 1 cup strawberry preserves with 1 thinly diced habanero pepper.

Grilled Burgers

PREP TIME: 20 minutes **COOK TIME:** 8 minutes **TOTAL TIME:** 28 minutes

Grilling is a great way to cook, especially in the warmer weather and for a bunch of people. One of the best things from the grill is a burger. Start with a clean, hot grill (it takes about 10 minutes to heat a gas grill and 15 minutes for charcoal to become white and ashy), wipe the grate with vegetable oil to prevent sticking, and, while it looks fancy to flip the food, resist; turning items increases the cooking time. Close the grill lid whenever possible while cooking to keep the grill at temperature. Remember to clean the grill when you're done (it is easier to clean while hot). **SERVES: 4**

1 pound ground beef

1 tablespoon
   steak seasoning

½ teaspoon salt

1 tablespoon vegetable oil

4 hamburger buns

APPLIANCE SWITCH-UP

TIP: To make stove-top burgers instead, heat 1 tablespoon vegetable oil in a large frying pan over medium-high heat for 2 minutes. Place the burger patties in the frying pan and cook for 3 minutes. You should see liquid in the frying pan. Don't press down on the patty while cooking, or you'll lose the flavorful juices. Flip and cook on the other side, based on how you like your meat cooked: 5 minutes for medium; 6 minutes for medium-well; 7 minutes for well-done.

1. Preheat the grill.

2. In a medium bowl, combine the ground beef, steak seasoning, and salt. Mix with your hands, and shape into 4 patties. Make an indentation on one side of each patty (this will help it remain flat as it cooks).

3. Brush the grill grates with the vegetable oil. Grill the patties, indentation-side up, for 5 minutes. Then, gently flip them over and grill 3 to 5 minutes more, until the hamburgers are done to your liking. Place on the buns.

REMIX TIPS:

→   Add a slice of cheese during the last minute of cooking, and close the grill to melt.

→   Top your burger with the traditional pickles, onion, mustard, and/or mayonnaise, or try topping it with a fried egg, mushrooms, avocado, macaroni and cheese, sliced pineapple, coleslaw, hummus, or peanut sauce. I've even seen folks swap the bun for glazed donuts.

→   If you prefer a toasted bun, open the bun and place the cut side on the grill for 7 to 10 seconds.

Queso Dip and Homemade Tortilla Chips

PREP TIME: 5 minutes   **COOK TIME:** 10 minutes   **TOTAL TIME:** 15 minutes

This Mexican-inspired cheese dip deserves only the best dipping chips, which is why you'll make your own. While your chips bake, start the queso so it all comes out at the same time. **MAKES: 1 CUP DIP AND 48 CHIPS**

For the tortilla chips

½ teaspoon ground cumin

½ teaspoon garlic powder

¼ teaspoon salt

2 tablespoons butter, melted

6 (7-inch) tortillas

For the queso dip

3 tablespoons butter

3 tablespoons all-purpose flour

¼ teaspoon salt

¼ teaspoon hot sauce

1 cup dairy, nut, or soy milk

½ cup shredded cheddar cheese

1. **To make the chips:** Preheat the oven to 400°F.

2. In a small bowl, combine the cumin, garlic powder, and salt. Brush butter over one side of each tortilla. Sprinkle the seasoning over each tortilla.

3. Make 2 stacks of 3 tortillas. Using a pizza cutter or paring knife, cut each stack into 8 triangles (cut in half lengthwise, then in half widthwise, then cut between each slice to create the 8 triangles).

4. Place the triangles in a single layer on an ungreased baking sheet on the center rack in the oven and bake for 9 minutes, or until lightly browned.

5. **To make the dip:** In a medium microwave-safe bowl, cook the butter in the microwave on high for 30 seconds, or until melted.

6. Stir in the flour, salt, hot sauce, milk, and cheddar cheese. Microwave on high for three 1-minute intervals, stirring at the end of each interval, or until the mixture thickens and bubbles.

REMIX TIPS:

→ Try adding diced jalapeño to the cheese sauce.

→ Experiment with different cheeses, like Colby, Pepper Jack, Monterey Jack, four-cheese blend, or other combinations of cheeses.

Pigs in a Blanket

PREP TIME: 10 minutes **COOK TIME:** 10 minutes **TOTAL TIME:** 20 minutes

Making your own hors d'oeuvres may seem intimidating, but do not let that stop you from trying this recipe—all it really requires is a little slicing and rolling to yield that perfect savory snack. So, grab those ingredients and crank up the toaster oven. This recipe serves six people, but even if you are alone, they have a way of disappearing. **SERVES: 6**

1 (8-ounce) can crescent roll dough

12 cocktail weenies

2 tablespoons butter, at room temperature

½ teaspoon salt

1. Preheat your toaster oven to 375°F. Line the toaster oven tray with aluminum foil.

2. Unroll the dough. There should be 8 rectangles of dough. Lay 4 of them on your work surface and pack up the rest for later (see Remix Tip).

3. Cut the 4 dough rectangles into 3 slender triangles each, then roll a cocktail weenie up inside each one.

4. Brush the rolled-up crescents with the softened butter, using your fingers to spread it evenly around the surface. Sprinkle each roll with salt.

5. Put the pigs in a blanket on the prepared tray and bake for 10 minutes, or until golden brown.

REMIX TIPS:

→ Separate the leftover dough between layers of wax paper, then wrap it in foil or plastic. Store it in the refrigerator for a few days, until you are ready to bake the rolls according to the package directions.

→ Add some flavor by spreading your favorite mustard or sprinkling a bit of cheese on the dough before you roll it up.

Slow Cooker Barbecue Sandwiches

PREP TIME: 5 minutes **COOK TIME:** 10 to 12 hours **TOTAL TIME:** 10 to 12 hours

I love this recipe because it makes really great pork barbecue sandwiches, but also because the slow cooker does all of the work. You can start at night, get a good night's sleep, and have it ready for the next day. Or start it in the morning, have a full day of classes and studying, and then finish it right before the party. **SERVES: 10 TO 12**

3 to 4 pounds pork shoulder

1 cup water, divided

1 medium onion, finely chopped

½ cup ketchup

2 tablespoons apple cider vinegar

1½ tablespoons Worcestershire sauce

1 tablespoon sugar

1 teaspoon Dijon mustard

1 teaspoon chili powder

1 teaspoon salt

10 to 12 Kaiser rolls or hamburger buns

1. The night before serving, put the pork shoulder in a slow cooker with ½ cup of water. Cover and cook on the low setting for 10 to 12 hours.

2. Also the night before serving, combine the onion, ketchup, vinegar, Worcestershire sauce, sugar, mustard, chili powder, salt, and the remaining ½ cup of water. Store in the refrigerator until the pork is done cooking.

3. In the morning, shred the pork with a fork and return it to the slow cooker. Pour the sauce over the pork and mix until well combined.

4. Heat on low until ready to serve. Serve on Kaiser rolls.

1 tablespoon sugar

1 tablespoon apple cider vinegar

¼ teaspoon salt

½ cup mayonnaise

1 (14-ounce) package coleslaw mix

REMIX TIP: In the South, barbecue pork is served topped with coleslaw, or you can serve it on the side. Here's how you make it:

1. In a small bowl, combine the sugar, vinegar, and salt, and whisk until sugar and salt are dissolved. Whisk in the mayonnaise until combined.

2. Put the coleslaw mix in a large mixing bowl. Add the mayonnaise mixture and toss until the coleslaw mix is evenly coated.

MAKE IT FASTER: To save a little time and for a more traditional take, skip making your own sauce and use a 28-ounce bottle of your favorite store-bought barbecue sauce instead.

Game Day Potato Salad

PREP TIME: 15 minutes **COOK TIME:** 7 minutes **TOTAL TIME:** 22 minutes

This "all-American" side dish, perfect for picnics, parties, and potlucks, actually came to the United States via German immigrants. The secret flare to this budget-friendly recipe is the pickle juice. Feel free to taste and season as you go. If you want it "wetter," add more mayonnaise and pickle juice. **SERVES: 6**

5 medium russet potatoes, peeled

½ cup mayonnaise

¼ cup thinly sliced celery

¼ cup chopped onion

¼ cup dill pickle juice

2 large dill pickles, finely chopped

2 hard-boiled eggs, sliced (pre-cooked or see Cobb Salad, page 60, for hard-boiling instructions)

1 tablespoon yellow mustard

1 teaspoon salt

½ teaspoon freshly ground black pepper

1. Prick each potato several times with a fork. Place potatoes 1 inch apart on a paper towel. Microwave on high for 7 minutes. Remove the potatoes from the microwave and let them rest for 5 minutes. Cut them into cubes or slices.

2. In a large mixing bowl, combine the mayonnaise, celery, onion, pickle juice, pickles, eggs, mustard, salt, and pepper. Mix until well combined.

3. Add the potatoes to the mayonnaise mixture and fold to coat the potatoes.

REMIX TIPS:

→ Make it your own by adding crumbled bacon, minced jalapeños, ½ teaspoon paprika, diced green chiles, relish, sliced banana peppers, or chopped scallions.

→ For a creamier egg potato salad, add 2 more hard-boiled eggs to the list of ingredients; mash the egg yolks into the mayonnaise mixture, then slice the egg whites and add them to the salad.

Walking Fish Nachos

PREP TIME: 9 minutes   **COOK TIME:** 6 minutes   **TOTAL TIME:** 15 minutes

Eat your nachos walking. These tantalizing treats will simply "walk" away from the table at your next party. They include all the goodness of a taco but in the palm of your hand. Bonus: The chip bag becomes the plate—what could be more convenient than that? **SERVES: 6**

1½ pounds tilapia fillets (about ½ inch thick)

2 tablespoons taco seasoning mix

½ teaspoon minced garlic

½ teaspoon ground cumin

½ cup chicken broth

1 large globe or beefsteak tomato, diced

4 snack-size bags of corn chips

Toppings of your choice: green chiles, shredded cheddar cheese, sour cream, sliced scallions, salsa, beans, fresh cilantro, black olives, hot sauce, etc.

1. In a microwave-safe baking dish, arrange fillets so the thicker parts are toward the outside of the dish. Sprinkle with the taco seasoning, garlic, and cumin. Add the chicken broth. Cover the dish with plastic wrap.

2. Microwave on high for 2 minutes, then rotate the fish. Repeat until the fish has cooked for 6 minutes, or until it flakes easily. Let rest for 5 minutes and drain any liquid from the dish.

3. Add the diced tomato and flake the fish to combine with the tomatoes.

4. When ready to serve, open a bag of corn chips. Add the fish mixture and any toppings you like. Use a fork and enjoy it direct from the bag.

REMIX TIP: Swap the fish for 1 pound of ground beef, shredded chicken, or pork, and follow these directions:

1. In a large frying pan over medium heat, combine the ground meat, cumin, and garlic. Cook, stirring continuously to break up the meat, for 6 minutes, or until the meat is no longer pink. Drain.

2. Add taco seasoning, diced tomatoes, and 1 (4-ounce) can green chiles, and stir until well mixed.

3. When ready to serve, open a bag of corn chips. Add the meat mixture and any toppings you like. Use a fork and enjoy direct from the bag.

Baked Chili Cheese Dogs

PREP TIME: 5 minutes **COOK TIME:** 40 minutes **TOTAL TIME:** 45 minutes

Invite some friends over to chill with these baked chili cheese dogs. A great game-day food, you can prep them and slide them into the oven when everyone arrives without having to fuss over them. You might want to have a backup tray or you'll be in the doghouse when they're gone in mere minutes. **SERVES: 8**

Nonstick cooking spray

8 hot dog buns

⅓ cup mayonnaise

¼ cup yellow mustard

8 kosher hot dogs

1 (10-ounce) can hot dog chili (or chili without beans)

1 cup chopped onions (optional)

2 chopped jalapeños (optional)

1½ cups shredded cheddar cheese

1. Preheat the oven to 350°F. Line a 9-by-13-inch baking pan with aluminum foil and spray it with cooking spray.

2. Open each of the hot dog buns and swipe mayonnaise and mustard on the inside of each one.

3. Place a hot dog in each bun. Cover the hot dogs with hot dog chili. Add onions and jalapeños (if using), and cover with the cheese.

4. Place aluminum foil over the hot dogs (make a tent, so the cheese does not stick to it).

5. Bake at 350°F for 40 minutes.

REMIX TIP: You can add sauerkraut, relish, coleslaw, or any of your favorite toppings to the hot dogs before covering with cheese and baking.

Pineapple Sausage Kebabs

PREP TIME: 15 minutes **COOK TIME:** 8 minutes **TOTAL TIME:** 23 minutes

Where people go wrong with kebabs is combining meats, vegetables, and fruits that all have different cooking times. This recipe uses ingredients that cook for the same amount of time: beef kielbasa (found with the deli meats), colorful veggies, and sweet pineapple. If you're using wooden kebab sticks, soak them in cold water for 30 minutes before starting to prevent them from burning or catching on fire. **SERVES: 4**

1 tablespoon vegetable oil

12 ounces beef kielbasa, or Polish sausage, sliced into rounds

1 red bell pepper, seeded and sliced

1 large zucchini, cut into ½-inch slices

1 fresh pineapple, peeled and cut into chunks

1 red onion, cut into 2-inch pieces

3 tablespoons pineapple juice

1 tablespoon soy sauce

½ cup Simple Barbecue Sauce (page 167)

1. Wipe the grill grates with the vegetable oil to prevent sticking, and preheat the grill.

2. Working with 1 kebab stick at a time, alternate kielbasa pieces, bell pepper slices, zucchini slices, pineapple chunks, and red onion pieces until each stick is full.

3. In a small bowl, combine the pineapple juice, soy sauce, and barbecue sauce.

4. Brush the kebabs with the sauce, saving half of it for basting during grilling.

5. Place the kebabs on the grill and cook for 4 minutes. Gently turn the kebabs over, brush sauce on them, and cook for 4 minutes more. Kebabs are done when the kielbasa is heated through and the vegetable edges are slightly charred.

APPLIANCE SWITCH-UP TIP: If you don't have grill access, preheat the oven to broil. Line a baking sheet with aluminum foil and spray it lightly with nonstick cooking spray. Skewer the kebabs and place them on the prepared baking sheet. Put the sheet on the top rack of the oven under the broiler for 5 minutes. Turn the kebabs and broil for 5 more minutes.

Turkey and Cheese Party Pinwheels

PREP TIME: 10 minutes, plus 30 minutes for chilling **TOTAL TIME:** 40 minutes

Pinwheels aren't just kids' toys. Turn your favorite sandwich into a fun appetizer sure to appeal to even your toughest foodie friends. The sky's the limit here: Try using ham, chorizo, roast beef, or pepperoni, and pair any of these meats with different cheeses. **MAKES: 12 PINWHEELS**

½ cup softened
   cream cheese

4 (10-inch)
   whole-wheat tortillas

1 avocado, peeled, pitted,
   and sliced (see Guaca-
   mole, Smart Shopping
   Tip, page 46, for how to
   choose an avocado)

½ pound sliced
   deli turkey

1 large Roma tomato,
   thinly sliced

4 romaine lettuce leaves,
   thinly sliced

8 slices Swiss cheese

1. Spread cream cheese over the tortillas evenly, leaving an inch of the tortilla uncovered at the edge.

2. Layer on the avocado, turkey, tomato, lettuce, and Swiss cheese.

3. Carefully roll up each tortilla, wrap in plastic wrap, and chill for at least 30 minutes before serving.

4. To serve, cut each tortilla crosswise into 3 increments to make 12 pinwheels.

REMIX TIPS:

→ Add the avocado to the cream cheese and use a hand mixer to beat until smooth before spreading it on the tortillas.

→ Spread the tortilla with 1 tablespoon pesto before or instead of adding the cream cheese.

→ Add sautéed onions or sautéed baby spinach to the tortillas before adding the turkey.

Tailgate Three-Bean Chili

PREP TIME: 10 minutes **COOK TIME:** 20 minutes **TOTAL TIME:** 30 minutes

Popular food lore traces chili's roots back to the 1800s in Texas. It was such a hit that the 1893 World's Fair in Chicago featured it in an exhibit called the San Antonio Chili Stand. This dish has stood the test of time; every family seems to have their own special recipe. Now you can, too. Make a pot of this tailgate chili for your next event, and you'll be sure to please the whole crowd. **SERVES: 4 TO 6**

3 tablespoons vegetable oil

1 cup finely sliced onion

¼ cup diced green bell pepper

3 tablespoons chili powder

¼ cup cold water

1 cup boiling water

1 cup canned tomato or vegetable juice

3 garlic cloves, minced

2 teaspoons sugar

½ teaspoon salt

2 (15-ounce) cans red kidney beans

1 (15-ounce) can pinto beans

1 (15-ounce) can black beans

1. In a large saucepan, warm the oil over medium-high heat for 1 minute. Add the onion and green pepper and cook for 5 minutes, or until the peppers are tender and the onion is translucent.

2. In a small bowl, combine the chili powder with the cold water and whisk to create a smooth paste. Set aside.

3. Add the boiling water and the tomato juice to the saucepan with the onions and green pepper, then whisk in the chili paste until well blended. Add the garlic, sugar, and salt.

4. Cover the saucepan with a lid, reduce the heat to medium-low, and simmer 10 minutes, or until heated through.

5. Add the beans and cook for 5 minutes, or until heated through.

REMIX TIPS:

→ If the chili gets too thick, add a tablespoon or two of hot water.

→ You can create even more distinctive flavor by adding ¼ cup strong espresso and 2 tablespoons unsweetened cocoa to the chili in step 3.

→ Serve with sour cream and grated cheddar cheese.

Baked Potato Skins

PREP TIME: 10 minutes **COOK TIME:** 50 minutes **TOTAL TIME:** 60 minutes

Crispy potato skins became trendy appetizers in restaurants in the 1970s, but they remain a party favorite today for good reason—especially when topped with melted cheese. If you're pressed for time, you can cook the potatoes in the microwave instead of in the oven. **SERVES: 4**

4 medium russet potatoes

1 tablespoon vegetable oil, plus extra for greasing the skillet

¼ teaspoon salt

½ cup shredded Pepper Jack or cheddar cheese

¼ cup chopped fresh chives

¼ cup plain Greek yogurt for dipping (optional)

....

REMIX TIP: To make these potato skins dairy-free, sprinkle them with nutritional yeast instead of using cheese. Top with diced avocado for a plant-based fat alternative, or dip potato skins in Guacamole (page 46) instead of Greek yogurt.

1. Preheat the oven to 450°F.

2. Score the potatoes with a fork, transfer them to a baking sheet, and bake for 30 minutes, or until you can easily pierce them with a fork.

3. Cool the potatoes for about 5 minutes, or until you can handle them comfortably. Slice them in half lengthwise and use a spoon to scoop out about half the potato flesh in each half. Reserve the scooped-out potato for another recipe, like Date-Night Steak and Mashed Potatoes (page 118).

4. Brush the potato skins with the vegetable oil and sprinkle with salt.

5. Lightly oil a large skillet set over medium heat. Arrange the scooped-out potatoes, cut-side down, in the skillet and cook for 15 minutes, or until the inside of the potato turns golden brown.

6. Flip the potatoes over, sprinkle with the cheese, and cook until the cheese is melted, about 3 minutes.

7. Top the potato skins with the chopped chives and serve with the yogurt for dipping (if using). Wrap any leftover potatoes in plastic wrap and refrigerate for up to 5 days.

Spinach and Artichoke Dip

PREP TIME: 5 minutes **COOK TIME:** 2 minutes **TOTAL TIME:** 7 minutes

This classic bar food is on appetizer menus throughout the country for good reason: It's seriously delicious. You can dip bread slices, veggie spears, or tortilla chips in it, use it as a base for flatbread, or even spread it as a condiment on your favorite sandwich. Feel free to get creative! It's easy to have around because this version takes under 10 minutes to make, start to finish. **SERVES: 4**

1 teaspoon canola oil

1 (15-ounce) can artichoke hearts, drained and roughly chopped

2 cups roughly chopped fresh spinach

2 garlic cloves, minced

8 ounces cream cheese, cut into 1-inch cubes

1 cup grated mozzarella cheese

½ teaspoon salt

¼ teaspoon freshly ground black pepper

1. In a microwave-safe dish, combine the oil, artichoke hearts, spinach, garlic, cream cheese, mozzarella, salt, and pepper. Microwave on high for 1 minute.

2. Stir, then microwave for 1 minute more, or until the cheese is melted.

REMIX TIP: Give it some heat by adding ¼ teaspoon hot sauce or ½ teaspoon red pepper flakes.

APPLIANCE SWITCH-UP TIP: Make this dip in the oven. Preheat the oven to 350° F. In a baking dish, layer the oil, artichoke hearts, spinach, garlic, cream cheese, and mozzarella cheese, and season with salt and pepper. Bake, uncovered, on the center rack for 20 minutes, or until the cheese is browned and bubbling. Stir before serving.

Barbecue Cauliflower Wings

PREP TIME: 10 minutes **COOK TIME:** 40 minutes **TOTAL TIME:** 50 minutes

No chicken? No problem. You won't even notice the cauliflower amid the sticky, messy, gooey, yummy tastiness of this recipe, but your body will; you'll just rake in the fiber and antioxidants. Your roomies will be begging for more. **SERVES: 4**

Extra-virgin olive
  oil, for coating the
  baking sheet

½ cup all-purpose flour

2 teaspoons
  garlic powder

Salt

Freshly ground
  black pepper

½ cup nondairy milk

¼ cup water

2 cups small
  cauliflower florets

½ cup Simple Barbecue
  Sauce (page 167)

½ cup Caesar dressing

1. Preheat the oven to 350°F. Coat a rimmed baking sheet with olive oil or line it with parchment paper or a silicone mat.

2. In a large bowl, combine the flour and garlic powder, and season to taste with salt and pepper. Whisk in the milk and water until thoroughly combined.

3. Dunk the cauliflower florets into the batter, ensuring they are fully coated, then put them on the prepared baking sheet in a single layer. Bake for 20 minutes.

4. Drizzle the cauliflower with barbecue sauce and carefully turn to coat. Bake for 20 minutes more.

5. Remove the cauliflower from the oven and let cool for a few minutes. Serve with Caesar dressing for dipping.

Bruschetta

PREP TIME: 11 minutes   **COOK TIME:** 4 minutes   **TOTAL TIME:** 15 minutes

In college I worked at an Italian restaurant where we served bruschetta (*bru-SKET-uh*) as an antipasto. The recipe is easy to replicate at home, will be widely popular, and is far less expensive than what most restaurants charge. It is also highly adaptable, so you can swap the tomatoes and basil for figs, goat cheese, and honey, or whatever sounds appetizing and is easy to access. **SERVES: 4**

1 pint grape or cherry tomatoes, halved

¼ cup roughly chopped fresh basil

2 tablespoons balsamic vinegar

½ teaspoon salt

¼ teaspoon freshly ground black pepper

8 slices crusty baguette

Nonstick cooking spray

1. In a small mixing bowl, combine the tomatoes, basil, and balsamic vinegar. Season with the salt and pepper. Set aside to allow the flavors to come together.

2. Preheat the toaster oven to 450°F and line the baking tray with foil. Spray the bread with cooking spray and put it in the toaster on the prepared tray. Cook for 2 minutes. Turn the bread over and cook for 2 more minutes, or until the bread is golden brown.

3. Top each of the bread slices with the tomato-basil mixture and serve immediately.

REMIX TIPS:

→ Try adding ¼ teaspoon red pepper flakes if you like it with a bit of heat.

→ Spread a little bit of garlic butter on the bread before toasting.

Home Team Sub Sandwich

PREP TIME: 15 minutes **TOTAL TIME:** 15 minutes

You might call this a hoagie (Philly), grinder (New England), hero (NYC), or sub, short for submarine (pockets all over the country). Whatever you call it can be sliced into individual servings for a bunch of guests. It will cut into sandwiches better if you allow it to chill for 1 hour in the refrigerator.

SERVES: 12

1 unsliced loaf Italian bread

¼ cup Italian dressing

¼ pound sliced deli roast beef

⅛ pound sliced provolone cheese

2 medium tomatoes, thinly sliced

⅛ pound thinly sliced salami

⅛ pound sliced cheddar cheese

½ head iceberg lettuce, finely chopped

¼ pound sliced deli chicken

1. Cut the loaf of bread lengthwise. Brush the insides of the bread with Italian dressing.

2. On the bottom side of the loaf, layer ingredients in this order: roast beef, provolone cheese, tomatoes, salami, cheddar cheese, lettuce, chicken. Drizzle with any remaining Italian dressing.

3. Add the top of the bread loaf. Serve immediately, or wrap tightly in plastic wrap and refrigerate before slicing.

REMIX TIP: For the best "fit," slightly hollow out the tops and bottoms of the loaf before layering ingredients.

MAKE IT YOURSELF TIP: Try making your own condiments and adding them to the sub:

→ For **honey mustard**, combine 2 tablespoons mayonnaise, 1 tablespoon yellow mustard, and ½ tablespoon honey.

→ For **cream cheese and chives**, combine 2 tablespoons cream cheese (at room temperature), 2 tablespoons sour cream, 1 teaspoon dried chives, ½ teaspoon dried minced onion, ⅛ teaspoon lemon pepper seasoning, and ¼ teaspoon garlic powder.

→ For **fry sauce**, combine ½ cup mayonnaise, 5 tablespoons ketchup, ½ teaspoon Worcestershire sauce, and ½ tablespoon pickle juice.

For each, combine all ingredients together in a small bowl and stir until well mixed.

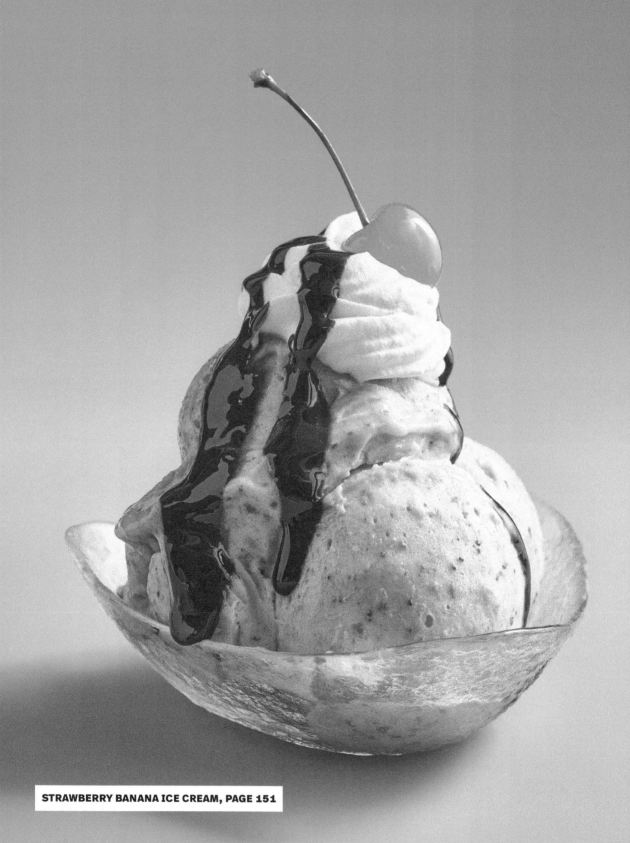

STRAWBERRY BANANA ICE CREAM, PAGE 151

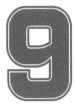

Desserts

Chocolate Pudding

PREP TIME: 5 minutes **COOK TIME:** 7 minutes **TOTAL TIME:** 12 minutes

When you find out how easy (and how much better-tasting) pudding from scratch is, you will never grab those preservative-filled pudding snack packs again. My children love this recipe, and it was a rite of passage when they could make it on their own. Now, it is their go-to when I tell them dessert isn't on my menu. **SERVES: 1**

1 tablespoon cornstarch

⅓ cup sugar

1 tablespoon unsweet-
ened cocoa powder

1 cup dairy, nut, or
soy milk

1 egg yolk (see Make It
Yourself Tip)

¼ teaspoon
vanilla extract

1 teaspoon butter

MAKE IT YOURSELF TIP:
To separate the egg yolk from the egg white, place a small bowl on your work space. Wash your hands. Crack the egg and gently pull the shell apart so you have two halves. Work the egg back and forth between the shells, letting the egg white fall into the small bowl, and keeping the yolk in the eggshell. You can also crack the egg and catch the yolk in your hand, letting the egg white fall through your fingers into the bowl.

1. In a medium saucepan over medium heat, combine the cornstarch, sugar, and cocoa. Whisk briefly to get any lumps out. Add the milk and whisk for 2 minutes. Add the egg yolk while whisking briskly.

2. Cook for 5 minutes, or until the mixture thickens. Be sure to stir constantly.

3. When the pudding has thickened, remove it from the heat. Add the vanilla and butter, and stir to incorporate.

4. Pour the pudding into a bowl and enjoy it warm or cover (see Remix Tip), let it cool for 15 minutes, and then move it to the refrigerator. The pudding will thicken more as it cools.

REMIX TIPS:

→ If you want to avoid a "skin" developing on top of the pudding, before refrigerating, cover it with plastic wrap and press down so that the wrap touches the pudding.

→ For vanilla pudding, omit the cocoa and add another ¼ teaspoon of vanilla extract.

→ For banana chocolate pudding, add ¼ teaspoon banana flavoring.

Apple Spice Mug Cake

PREP TIME: 5 minutes **COOK TIME:** 2 minutes **TOTAL TIME:** 7 minutes

Satisfy that sweet tooth in 7 minutes or less. There's no need to make an entire cake when you can make one serving and eat it straight from your favorite mug. For variety, change out the apple spice for pumpkin spice, cinnamon, sprinkles, or cocoa, and have yourself a mug cake for every day of the week. **SERVES: 1**

2 tablespoons butter

¼ cup all-purpose flour

2 tablespoons sugar

1 teaspoon apple pie spice

¼ teaspoon baking powder

⅛ teaspoon salt

1 egg yolk, beaten (see Chocolate Pudding, Make It Yourself Tip, page 142)

1 tablespoon dairy, nut, or soy milk

1 teaspoon vanilla extract

1. In an 8-ounce microwave-safe mug, spoon in the butter and microwave for 10 seconds, or until melted. Add the flour, sugar, apple pie spice, baking powder, and salt. Stir until well mixed. Add the egg yolk, milk, and vanilla, and stir until the mixture is smooth.

2. Microwave on high for 1 minute 30 seconds, or until the top of the "cake" pulls away from the mug. Allow to rest for 1 minute before eating.

REMIX TIP: Make it a true celebration by drizzling it with caramel sauce, topping it with Homemade Whipped Cream (page 165), adding your favorite frosting, or serving with ice cream.

Cake S'mores

PREP TIME: 5 minutes **COOK TIME:** 15 seconds **TOTAL TIME:** 6 minutes

You don't have time *not* to make this dessert. Bring back the old camp days with this campfire-classic-turned-cake, and you'll be wishing you were in a tent under the stars. **SERVES: 1**

2 slices pound cake

2 tablespoons miniature marshmallows

2 tablespoons chocolate chips

1. Put the cake slices on a microwave-safe plate. Evenly distribute the marshmallows and chocolate chips on top of the cake slices.

2. Place the plate in the microwave and heat on high for 15 seconds, or until the marshmallows puff up. Let it rest for 10 seconds, then eat as is or place one slice on top of the other to make a s'mores sandwich.

REMIX TIPS:

→ Add caramel topping, nuts, or Homemade Whipped Cream (page 165).

→ If you want more "toasted" marshmallows, put them under a broiler for 2 minutes, or until the marshmallows are golden.

→ Try replacing the pound cake with graham crackers for a more traditional s'more experience.

Angel Food Cream Pie

PREP TIME: 10 minutes **COOK TIME:** 30 seconds **TOTAL TIME:** 11 minutes

In just a few minutes, you can create my take on the traditional Boston cream pie. It features layers of angel food cake with creamy vanilla custard, topped with decadent chocolate frosting. You're about to become the most popular person on your floor. **SERVES: 10**

1 (1-ounce) box instant vanilla pudding

1½ cups cold dairy, nut, or soy milk

1 (10- to 14-ounce) bakery angel food cake, Bundt style (or see Make It Yourself Tip)

1 (16-ounce) container chocolate frosting

1. In a small mixing bowl, whisk the instant pudding with cold milk until thickened.

2. Slice the angel food cake, horizontally, into 3 even layers.

3. Spread pudding evenly among the 3 angel food cake layers, stacking each layer one on top of the other.

4. Heat the container of chocolate frosting in the microwave for 30 seconds.

5. Stir the warmed chocolate frosting and then pour it over the layered angel food cake. The frosting will set as it cools.

REMIX TIP: Add sliced strawberries on top of the pudding between each layer of angel food cake.

MAKE IT YOURSELF TIP: Use 1 (16-ounce) box of angel food cake mix and follow the package instructions. Allow the cake to cool completely, and then begin the recipe.

Party Popcorn

PREP TIME: 5 minutes **COOK TIME:** 15 minutes **TOTAL TIME:** 20 minutes

Who doesn't love popcorn? This recipe takes the traditional snack and turns it into caramel corn. Shape it into balls or add your favorite toppings. I have included three of my favorite mixes below, but let your imagination run wild. Are you looking for savory? Try adding rice cereal, pretzels, or bacon. For a sweet version, small bite-size candies work great (think mini peanut butter cups). **SERVES: 1 (WITH LOTS OF LEFTOVERS)**

8 cups popped popcorn

1⅓ cups sugar

1 cup butter

½ cup light corn syrup

1 teaspoon vanilla extract

1. Pour the popcorn onto a baking sheet.

2. In a medium saucepan set over medium heat, combine the sugar, butter, corn syrup, and vanilla. Boil for 10 to 15 minutes, or until it reaches a light caramel color. Pour the mixture over the popcorn, mix to coat the popcorn evenly, and spread it out to dry for about 10 minutes.

REMIX TIPS:

→ Nut Crunch: Add 1⅓ cup chopped pecans and ⅔ cup sliced almonds.

→ Cranberry Marshmallow: Add 2 cups miniature marshmallows, 1 cup dried cranberries, 1 cup chopped walnuts, and 2 tablespoons grated orange peel.

→ Bacon Crunch: Sprinkle 1 cup crumbled crisp bacon over the popcorn.

→ If you don't have corn syrup, use honey or maple syrup in its place.

No-Bake Power Bites

PREP TIME: 10 minutes **TOTAL TIME:** 10 minutes

These no-bake protein bites are a great pre-workout, pre-study, post-study, or midnight no-guilt snack. They are super easy to make, and you can store them in an airtight container in the refrigerator so they're ready to snack on. The protein powder can be any flavor and any brand. Shop around to find your favorite. **MAKES: 12 BITES**

1½ cups old-fashioned oats

1 cup nut butter

¼ cup honey

4 tablespoons protein powder

In a large bowl, combine the oats, nut butter, honey, and protein powder. Mix until moist and able to form balls (slightly less moist than cookie dough). If the mixture is too dry, add water, 1 tablespoon at a time, being careful not to make it too moist. Shape the mixture into 1½-inch balls and eat, or refrigerate for up to 1 week.

REMIX TIPS:

→ Roll balls in coconut, cocoa, or chopped nuts.

→ Stir in ¼ cup raisins or other dried fruit, chocolate chips, chopped nuts, or seeds.

Fruit Crisp

PREP TIME: 5 minutes **COOK TIME:** 30 minutes **TOTAL TIME:** 35 minutes

Fruit crisp is a classic comfort dessert. You can swap the peaches for berries, cherries, or any fruity combination. It tastes best warm from the oven. This fruit crisp is delicious as is, but you can add a scoop of vanilla ice cream or dollop of Homemade Whipped Cream (page 165) to take it up a notch. **SERVES: 1**

½ cup sliced peaches, drained (canned, fresh and peeled, or frozen)

1½ teaspoons quick oats (not instant)

1½ teaspoons all-purpose flour

¾ teaspoon packed brown sugar

1¼ teaspoons cold butter

¼ teaspoon vanilla extract

1. Preheat the oven to 375°F.

2. In a 6-ounce baking dish, spread out the sliced peaches.

3. In a small bowl, combine the oats, flour, and brown sugar, and stir to combine. Using 2 forks, cut the butter into the mixture until it looks like coarse crumbs. Add the vanilla and sprinkle over the peaches.

4. Bake on the center rack for 30 minutes, or until it bubbles. Serve warm or cold.

APPLIANCE SWITCH-UP TIP: To use the microwave instead of the oven, cover the baking dish with wax paper and cook on high for 6 minutes.

Chocolate Coconut Bars

PREP TIME: 23 minutes **COOK TIME:** 2 minutes **TOTAL TIME:** 25 minutes

With their coconut base, these bars are not only so much more delicious than store-bought bars, but they are also quite filling. Fat from the coconut oil can increase HDL (good) cholesterol and help with hormone and gut-flora balance. But because these bars are bound with coconut oil, they do need to stay refrigerated to hold their shape. If vegan isn't your thing, feel free to sub in regular semisweet chocolate chips. **MAKES: 16 BARS**

¼ cup coconut oil or unsalted vegan margarine, plus more to grease baking dish

2 cups unsweetened shredded coconut

¼ cup sugar

2 tablespoons simple syrup or maple syrup

1 cup vegan chocolate chips

1. Coat an 8-by-8-inch baking dish with coconut oil (or line it with parchment paper) and set aside.

2. In a small mixing bowl, stir together the coconut oil, shredded coconut, sugar, and syrup. Transfer the mixture to the prepared baking dish and press it down firmly with the back of a spoon.

3. In a small microwave-safe bowl, heat the chocolate chips on high for 1 minute. Stir. Continue heating in 30-second increments, stirring after each, until the chocolate is melted. Pour and spread the melted chocolate over the coconut base and let it sit until the chocolate hardens, about 20 minutes.

4. Cut into 16 bars. They will keep, covered and refrigerated, for up to 1 week.

White Chocolate and Lime Mini Cheesecakes

PREP TIME: 10 minutes, plus 4 hours to chill **TOTAL TIME:** 4 hours 10 minutes

This dessert is delicious, simple to make, and totally worth the chill time. It makes a brilliant treat to share at the end of the day with roommates or five lucky guests. Don't forget to take your butter and cream cheese out of the fridge in advance to give them a chance to reach room temperature. **SERVES: 6**

For the crust

Nonstick cooking spray

¾ cup crushed graham crackers (from 8 graham cracker squares)

3 tablespoons unsalted butter, at room temperature

1 tablespoon sugar

For the filling

12 ounces cream cheese, at room temperature

3 tablespoons lime juice

½ teaspoon lime zest

¼ cup sugar

½ teaspoon vanilla extract

½ cup Homemade Whipped Cream (page 165)

3 tablespoons white chocolate chips

1. **To make the crust:** Line a 6-cup muffin tin with cupcake liners, or place liners on a baking sheet. Lightly spray them with cooking spray. In a small mixing bowl, mix the graham crackers, butter, and sugar until combined.

2. Spoon the crust mixture, evenly divided, into the prepared muffin tin and press it down gently.

3. **To make the filling:** In the same bowl, combine the cream cheese, lime juice, lime zest, sugar, and vanilla to create a smooth mixture.

4. Once smooth, mix in the whipped cream and white chocolate chips, then divide and spoon it evenly into the crust in the muffin tin.

5. Cover and refrigerate for at least 4 hours to allow the mixture to become firm.

REMIX TIP: For a smoother texture, use a microwave to melt the white chocolate before mixing it in.

Strawberry Banana Ice Cream

PREP TIME: 5 minutes **TOTAL TIME:** 5 minutes

When you have extra bananas that are starting to turn brown, slice and spread them in a single layer on a freezer-safe plate or baking sheet and stick them in the freezer. The next day, transfer the banana slices to a resealable bag and store them in the freezer for up to three months. Frozen bananas are ideal for smoothies, but you can also use them to make a fruity alternative to store-bought ice cream. It is similar to the texture of soft-serve ice cream but so much more nutritious, and you can make it in just a few minutes with a blender or food processor. **SERVES: 2**

2 cups frozen banana slices (about 4 small bananas)

1 cup frozen strawberries

¼ cup dairy, soy, or nut milk, or more as needed

⅛ teaspoon salt

In a blender, combine the bananas, strawberries, milk, and salt, and blend for 1 minute, or until smooth and creamy, scraping down the sides with a spatula as needed. If the mixture is not blending well, add a little more milk and process again. The blend should be the consistency of soft-serve ice cream. Serve immediately with any toppings desired.

REMIX TIP: Frozen bananas provide the creamy, cool texture for this treat, but you can add all sorts of ingredients to change the flavor. Try cocoa powder, peanut butter, pitted cherries, or even matcha. Add any toppings you usually like to have on ice cream sundaes, like whipped cream, chocolate sauce, sprinkles, maraschino cherries, or chopped nuts.

Snickerdoodle Skillet Cookie

PREP TIME: 20 minutes **COOK TIME:** 20 minutes **TOTAL TIME:** 40 minutes

If you want to become the go-to room in your dorm, just start baking this aromatic recipe and the company won't stop coming. Mix this cinnamon-spiced cookie dough in one bowl and bake it in a single skillet. Serve the cookie right out of the pan or slice it into wedges. Freshly baked, it has a crispy outside and chewy inside, so you get the best of both cookie worlds. **SERVES: 8**

Nonstick cooking spray

½ cup packed
  brown sugar

½ cup granulated sugar,
  plus extra for topping

¼ cup (½ stick)
  butter, melted

1 tablespoon ground
  cinnamon, plus extra
  for topping

1 large egg

1 teaspoon vanilla extract

1 cup all-purpose flour

¼ teaspoon baking soda

1. Preheat the oven to 375°F. Spray a 10-inch oven-safe (cast iron or stainless steel) skillet with cooking spray.

2. In a large bowl, stir together the brown sugar, granulated sugar, melted butter, and cinnamon until there are no large lumps.

3. Add the egg and vanilla, stirring to combine. Add the flour and baking soda and stir until a thick dough forms. Use your hands to mix at the end, if needed.

4. Press the dough firmly into the greased skillet and sprinkle with additional granulated sugar and cinnamon, if desired.

5. Bake the skillet cookie for 20 minutes, or until the edges are golden and the center is baked through. Allow the cookie to cool, 15 to 20 minutes. Then slice it in the skillet, or flip the skillet over to release the cookie and slice it into 8 wedges. You can wrap the cookie in plastic or beeswax wrap and store it in an airtight container at room temperature for up to 1 week.

REMIX TIPS:

→ Make the dough into individual cookies by using a spoon and your hands to create dough balls. Place the balls on a parchment-lined baking or toaster sheet about 2 inches apart, and bake for 8 minutes at 350° F, or until the edges are lightly browned and the centers are still glossy.

→ Instead of cinnamon, try swapping in ½ cup chocolate chips. During the fall months, replace the cinnamon with pumpkin pie spice, which is made with cinnamon but also contains other warming spices, like ginger, nutmeg, and cloves.

Three-Ingredient Nut-Butter Brownies

PREP TIME: 10 minutes **COOK TIME:** 20 minutes **TOTAL TIME:** 30 minutes

Everyone needs a go-to brownie recipe. After all, warm brownies are the perfect motivator for study sessions, accompaniment for TV binges, and dessert when entertaining friends. This recipe uses just three ingredients for delicious, moist, melt-in-your-mouth brownies. And with no added sugar and lots of protein, they are even good for you. **SERVES: 8 TO 12**

Nonstick cooking spray

1 cup nut butter (like peanut, almond, or cashew)

2 eggs

¾ cup all-purpose flour

1. Preheat the oven to 350°F. Grease an 8-by-8-inch baking pan with cooking spray.

2. In a medium bowl, combine the nut butter, eggs, and flour. Mix until you have a thick, shiny, smooth batter. Make sure there are no lumps.

3. Pour the batter into the prepared pan.

4. Place on the center rack of the oven and bake for 20 minutes, or until a toothpick inserted in the center comes out clean.

REMIX TIPS:

→ Add ¼ cup chopped walnuts to the batter.

→ When cool, sift powdered sugar over the top or ice it with chocolate frosting.

Deep-Dish Microwave Cookie

PREP TIME: 8 minutes **COOK TIME:** 2 minutes **TOTAL TIME:** 10 minutes

You know those deep-dish skillet cookies often served at chain restaurants with a scoop of ice cream on top? The ones with the crisp edges and chewy, gooey center? Now you can make your own in no time flat. Just mix in all the right ingredients and— voilà!—your very own deep-dish cookie. **SERVES: 1**

1 tablespoon
  unsalted butter

2 tablespoons packed
  light brown sugar

1 tablespoon vanilla
  Greek yogurt

⅛ teaspoon
  vanilla extract

¼ cup all-purpose flour

¼ teaspoon
  baking powder

⅛ teaspoon salt

2 tablespoons semisweet
  chocolate chips

1. Put the butter in a large microwave-safe bowl and microwave for 20 to 25 seconds, or until melted.

2. Add the brown sugar, yogurt, and vanilla, and stir to combine.

3. Add the flour, baking powder, and salt, and stir to combine. Fold in the chocolate chips until evenly mixed.

4. Microwave for 40 to 45 seconds. Let the cookie rest 10 to 15 seconds before using a toothpick to check the center. If it is covered in raw batter, microwave for 10 to 15 seconds more. If the toothpick is clean or has just a few crumbs, the cookie is ready to enjoy.

REMIX TIP: For a flavor change, try butterscotch chips.

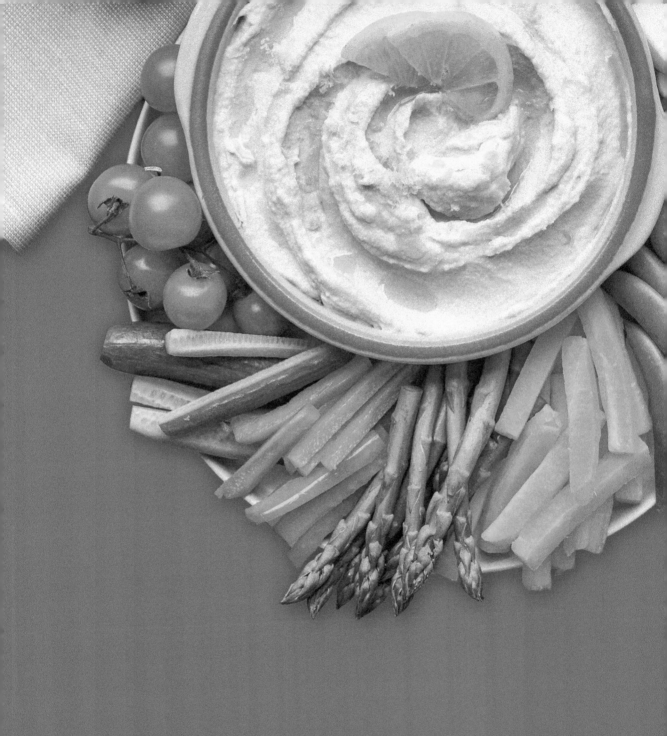

HUMMUS, PAGE 166

10

Staples

20-Second Homemade Mayonnaise

PREP TIME: 5 minutes **TOTAL TIME:** 5 minutes

Mayonnaise is a common staple in so many recipes. It can be used as a sandwich spread, as part of a sauce, or as an ingredient in potato salad. It's easy to make with a blender and just four ingredients. This quick homemade version tastes so much better than store-bought, you may never go back. **MAKES: 1⅓ CUPS**

1 egg

2 tablespoons lemon juice

¼ teaspoon salt

1 cup vegetable oil, divided

1. In a blender bowl, combine the egg, lemon juice, salt, and ¼ cup of oil. Cover and blend on medium-low for 10 seconds.

2. Open the pour spout (or remove the inner cap from the lid) and, while blending on medium, quickly add the remaining ¾ cup of oil. This addition and blending should take about 10 seconds. Store in an airtight container in the refrigerator for up to 3 days.

REMIX TIPS:

→ Add ½ teaspoon dry mustard for more flavor in the mayo.

→ For a healthier version, follow the same directions using ¼ cup plus 2 tablespoons extra-virgin olive oil instead of the vegetable oil and using 1 tablespoon lemon juice instead of 2. If you want it tangier, add more lemon juice.

Easy Salsa

PREP TIME: 10 minutes **TOTAL TIME:** 10 minutes

Salsa reportedly overtook ketchup as the number 1 selling condiment in the United States in the 1990s. And it's no wonder: With all of the varieties, this fresh and spicy sauce, perfect for dipping or topping, is healthy (it was officially designated a vegetable by the Department of Agriculture in 1998!) and flavorful. Our favorite twist is adding chopped avocado into the mix. **MAKES: 2½ CUPS**

2 cups Roma tomatoes

½ cup minced cilantro leaves (optional)

¼ cup diced white onion

2 tablespoons lemon juice

½ teaspoon minced garlic

1 teaspoon salt

¾ teaspoon ground cumin

In a medium mixing bowl, combine the tomatoes, cilantro (if using), onion, lemon juice, garlic, salt, and cumin. Serve immediately or refrigerate in an airtight container for up to 4 days.

REMIX TIP: Consider these add-ins (or any others you think sound good): jalapeño, chopped bell pepper, chopped avocado, chopped mango.

Lemon Curd

PREP TIME: 10 minutes **COOK TIME:** 5 minutes **TOTAL TIME:** 15 minutes

This delectable, literally mouthwatering lemon curd makes an excellent topping or filling. It is delicious stirred into plain yogurt. You can use it to fill a pie or layer on cakes (try it in the Angel Food Cream Pie, page 145). It can even elevate plain old toast. And don't underestimate the deliciousness of a spoonful all on its own. **MAKES: 2 CUPS**

3 tablespoons unsalted butter, melted

⅓ cup sugar

1 large egg

1 teaspoon lemon zest

⅓ cup lemon juice

⅛ teaspoon salt

1. In a small microwave-safe bowl, melt the butter in 30-second increments in the microwave on high, and then add the sugar, egg, lemon zest and juice, and salt, and whisk until smooth.

2. Microwave on high for 1 minute. Stir the mixture and microwave for 1 more minute. Let it stand in the microwave for 2 minutes and then whisk briskly.

3. Microwave for another 30 seconds. Let it stand for 3 minutes, and then whisk again. Take a spoon and scrape through the curd, making a "ditch." If the "ditch" fills with curd, microwave another 30 seconds, let stand for 2 minutes, and repeat. When the "ditch" remains, the curd is done.

4. Store the curd in an airtight container in the refrigerator, and use within 5 days.

REMIX TIPS:

→ To make a berry curd instead of lemon curd, use a fruit puree or fruit juice in place of lemon juice.

→ To make lemon curd mousse, fold ¾ cup lemon curd into ¾ cup whipped cream. Place ¼ cup curd in the bottom of a dessert glass, spoon in the curd-and-whipped-cream mixture, and top with ¼ cup whipped cream. Garnish with a lemon slice or vanilla wafer.

Trail Mix

PREP TIME: 5 minutes **TOTAL TIME:** 5 minutes

My dad loves the outdoors, and my children all came to associate Grandpa with trail mix. As they grew up, they learned to make it themselves for their outdoor adventures, movie nights, and study sessions. It's a nutritious and tasty takeaway, and a filling protein boost that you can customize to whatever you have on hand and to your mood. **MAKES: 4½ CUPS**

¾ cup chopped dried fruit

¾ cup roasted cashews

¾ cup roasted peanuts

¾ cup roasted almonds

½ cup candy-coated chocolates

½ cup semisweet chocolate chips

¼ cup toasted pumpkin seeds

¼ cup toasted coconut

In a gallon-size resealable bag, combine the dried fruit, cashews, peanuts, almonds, candy-coated chocolates, chocolate chips, pumpkin seeds, and coconut, and shake until thoroughly mixed.

REMIX TIP: You can add mini pretzels, rice cereal, or even mix roasted salted nuts with honey-roasted nuts for a sweet and savory blend.

Traditional Granola

PREP TIME: 10 minutes **COOK TIME:** 20 minutes **TOTAL TIME:** 30 minutes

Granola is a staple that you'll reach for multiple times a day. Delicious by the handful as a snack, it can also form the basis of a nutritious and filling breakfast as cereal or added to yogurt. It also provides that perfect crunch when used as an ice cream topper. If you're strapped for time, try the Quick Toaster Oven Granola (page 163). **MAKES: 6 CUPS**

Nonstick cooking spray

½ cup packed light brown sugar

½ cup honey

¼ cup olive or coconut oil

3 cups quick oats (not instant)

1½ cups chopped walnuts

1 cup slivered almonds

1 cup cashews

1 cup shredded sweet coconut

1 teaspoon salt

1 cup dried fruit, like raisins, cranberries, apricots, dates, or a combination

1. Preheat the oven to 300°F. Lay out parchment paper (or aluminum foil lightly sprayed with cooking spray) on a baking sheet.

2. In a medium bowl, combine the brown sugar, honey, and oil, and whisk until the sugar is dissolved, about 3 minutes.

3. Add the oats, walnuts, almonds, cashews, coconut, and salt to the oil mixture, and stir to coat.

4. Pour onto the prepared baking sheet, and spread with a spatula into an even layer.

5. Place on the center rack of the oven, and bake for 20 minutes, or until golden brown.

6. Sprinkle the hot granola with dried fruit and allow to cool before eating or storing. This granola can be stored in an airtight container on a shelf or in the refrigerator for up to 2 weeks.

Quick Toaster Oven Granola

PREP TIME: 5 minutes **COOK TIME:** 15 minutes **TOTAL TIME:** 20 minutes

MAKES: 1½ CUPS

Nonstick cooking spray

¾ cups quick oats
(not instant)

¼ cup slivered almonds
(or other nuts)

¼ cup shredded
sweet coconut

¼ teaspoon salt

2 tablespoons light
brown sugar

2 tablespoons
maple syrup

1 tablespoon melted
coconut oil or
extra-virgin olive oil

1. Preheat the toaster oven to 325°F and spray cooking spray on the toaster tray.

2. In a medium bowl, mix together the oats, nuts, coconut, and salt.

3. In a small bowl, whisk together the brown sugar, maple syrup, and oil.

4. Pour the brown sugar mixture over the oat mixture and stir to coat all the ingredients.

5. Pour the granola mixture onto the prepared tray and use a spatula to evenly spread it out.

6. Place the tray in the toaster oven and bake for 7 minutes. Stir the granola, moving the granola in the center to the edges and granola near the edges to the center, to bake evenly. Bake 7 more minutes, or until the granola is golden. (Watch carefully in the last few minutes to prevent the granola from burning.)

7. Remove the tray from the toaster oven and allow granola to cool without stirring.

REMIX TIPS:

→ Use different nuts like peanuts or pecans.

→ Try dark brown sugar instead of light brown sugar to bring out a more molasses or dark caramel flavor.

Basic Vinaigrette

PREP TIME: 5 minutes **TOTAL TIME:** 5 minutes

If you have a basic vinaigrette in your arsenal, you will always have salad dressing on hand and will never have to resort to those sugary store-bought varieties. Plus, this vinaigrette is so versatile, it can be used for a marinade or a sandwich enhancer as well. **MAKES: ¾ CUP**

½ cup extra-virgin olive oil

3 tablespoons vinegar, your choice (see Remix Tip)

1 tablespoon Dijon mustard

1 tablespoon sugar

2 garlic cloves, minced

¼ teaspoon salt

⅛ teaspoon freshly ground black pepper

In a small mixing bowl (or salad dressing bottle), combine the oil, vinegar, mustard, sugar, garlic, salt, and pepper, and whisk (or shake) the until sugar dissolves. Store the dressing for up to 2 weeks in the refrigerator in an airtight container.

REMIX TIP: The type of vinegar you use will change the flavor profile. Red wine vinegar will give it a bold flavor to pick up the flavors of tomatoes, bell peppers, etc. White wine vinegar is more mellow for cucumbers and spring greens. Apple cider vinegar is sweet and tangy, while balsamic is tart and tangy.

Homemade Whipped Cream

PREP TIME: 5 minutes **TOTAL TIME:** 5 minutes

Homemade whipped cream is too easy and too good to pass up. It's so much better than what you can buy in a store. Whip up a batch for coffee, a dessert topping, waffles, pancakes; mix with pudding or curd for fluffy mousse; or fold fruit into it for a fruit salad. It has so many possibilities. **MAKES: 2 CUPS**

1 cup heavy (whipping) cream

1 tablespoon powdered sugar

1 teaspoon vanilla extract

1. In a large mixing bowl, combine the heavy cream, powdered sugar, and vanilla.

2. Whisk by hand or with a hand mixer on medium speed until medium peaks form, about 4 minutes. When you lift the whisk or beaters from the whipped cream, medium peaks will hold their shape well: The tip of the peak curls over on itself, and the peak will droop but not disappear. Don't overmix or you'll have butter. And eat it quickly, because it will only last a day or two in the refrigerator.

REMIX TIPS:

→ The colder the cream, the easier it will whip. Colder cream makes the lightest whipped cream. Try putting a stainless-steel mixing bowl in the freezer for 15 to 30 minutes before starting for best results.

→ Add flavored syrups in place of vanilla to create flavored whipped cream.

Hummus

PREP TIME: 10 minutes **TOTAL TIME:** 10 minutes

Hummus is such a crowd-pleaser, it's great to have your own variety to bring to the party. It's also nice to keep around the dorm room because it is such a good source of complex carbohydrates, healthy fats, and plant-based protein. Plus, there are so many ways to create twists on hummus by adding items to the mix, like caramelized onions, pesto, or cilantro. I've even seen (though not tried) chocolate hummus. **MAKES: 1 CUP**

1 (15-ounce) can chickpeas, drained and rinsed

¼ cup tahini

1 garlic clove

3 tablespoons lemon juice

2 tablespoons extra-virgin olive oil, plus more for drizzling

¼ teaspoon salt

In a blender bowl, combine the chickpeas, tahini, garlic, lemon juice, 2 tablespoons olive oil, and salt. Puree until smooth and drizzle with olive oil. Store covered in the refrigerator for up to 3 days.

REMIX TIP: Make it a roasted red pepper hummus by adding 1 cup roughly chopped roasted red peppers to the recipe and blending until smooth.

Simple Barbecue Sauce

PREP TIME: 5 minutes **COOK TIME:** 1 to 7 minutes **TOTAL TIME:** 6 to 12 minutes

Especially in the American South, making barbecue sauce is something of an art, and definitely a point of pride. So, yes, you can buy barbecue sauce, but why not join in the craft and make your own from this simple recipe? You may not choose to enter a barbecue sauce competition, but you will know what's in your food. Heating the sauce is optional, so you can still make this if you don't have a stove or microwave, but briefly cooking it does bring the flavors together better. **MAKES: 1 CUP**

⅔ cup ketchup (see Make It Yourself Tip)

⅓ cup apple cider vinegar

¼ cup packed brown sugar

2 tablespoons soy sauce or tamari

¼ teaspoon garlic powder

⅛ teaspoon red pepper flakes

1. **On the stove top or hot plate:** In a medium saucepan, stir together the ketchup, vinegar, brown sugar, soy sauce, garlic powder, and red pepper flakes. Bring to a simmer over medium-low heat and cook for 5 minutes.

2. **In the microwave:** In a microwave-safe bowl, stir together the ketchup, vinegar, brown sugar, soy sauce, garlic powder, and red pepper flakes, cover, and heat on high for 1 minute.

3. Let cool. Store in an airtight container in the refrigerator for up to 1 week.

REMIX TIP: Add 1 to 2 teaspoons smoked paprika and/or a few drops of liquid smoke for a smoky flavor.

MAKE IT YOURSELF TIP: To make your own ketchup, in a small saucepan, combine 3 tablespoons tomato paste, 1 tablespoon sugar, 2 tablespoons distilled white vinegar, 1 tablespoon water, ¼ teaspoon sugar, ⅛ teaspoon salt, ¼ teaspoon onion powder, and ¼ teaspoon garlic powder over medium heat. Whisk until the sugar dissolves. Cook for 5 minutes, or until the sauce thickens to the desired consistency.

Latte

PREP TIME: 2 minutes **COOK TIME:** 30 seconds **TOTAL TIME:** 3 minutes

Skip the pricey coffee shop and make lattes at home. Whereas a traditional latte is a combination of steamed milk and espresso, the Remix Tips offer other options beyond plain coffee. Whether it starts your day or ends your day, it is a delicious warm drink that you will look forward to drinking. Experiment with flavors and make it your way. **SERVES: 1**

1 cup dairy, nut, or
  soy milk

1 teaspoon honey

¾ cup strong coffee

1. In a small microwave-safe mug, combine the milk and honey, and microwave for 30 seconds.

2. Whisk the warmed milk vigorously for 30 seconds to create a foam.

3. Pour the coffee into the foam.

REMIX TIPS:

→ Create your own caramel latte simply by adding 1 teaspoon caramel topping.

→ For these three varieties, prepare as above but omit the coffee and add the ingredients to ¾ cup hot water:

Turmeric: ¼ teaspoon ground turmeric and ⅛ teaspoon freshly ground black pepper

Matcha: 1 teaspoon matcha

Ginger: ¼ teaspoon ground ginger and 1 additional teaspoon honey

Measurement Conversions

Volume Equivalents (Liquid)

US STANDARD	US STANDARD (OUNCES)	METRIC (APPROXIMATE)
2 tablespoons	1 fl. oz.	30 mL
¼ cup	2 fl. oz.	60 mL
½ cup	4 fl. oz.	120 mL
1 cup	8 fl. oz.	240 mL
1½ cups	12 fl. oz.	355 mL
2 cups or 1 pint	16 fl. oz.	475 mL
4 cups or 1 quart	32 fl. oz.	1 L
1 gallon	128 fl. oz.	4 L

Oven Temperatures

FAHRENHEIT	CELSIUS (APPROXIMATE)
250°F	120°C
300°F	150°C
325°F	165°C
350°F	180°C
375°F	190°C
400°F	200°C
425°F	220°C
450°F	230°C

Volume Equivalents (Dry)

US STANDARD	METRIC (APPROXIMATE)
⅛ teaspoon	0.5 mL
¼ teaspoon	1 mL
½ teaspoon	2 mL
¾ teaspoon	4 mL
1 teaspoon	5 mL
1 tablespoon	15 mL
¼ cup	59 mL
⅓ cup	79 mL
½ cup	118 mL
⅔ cup	156 mL
¾ cup	177 mL
1 cup	235 mL
2 cups or 1 pint	475 mL
3 cups	700 mL
4 cups or 1 quart	1 L

Weight Equivalents

US STANDARD	METRIC (APPROXIMATE)
½ ounce	15 g
1 ounce	30 g
2 ounces	60 g
4 ounces	115 g
8 ounces	225 g
12 ounces	340 g
16 ounces or 1 pound	455 g

Index

Acknowledgments

Writing a book is humbling and rewarding. It's back-to-back deadlines in a short span of time. I have an amazing core group who have helped this dream of mine bloom.

None of this would have been possible without my family.

To my husband, thank you for stepping up when we rescued Molly Pop! And 60 days later (in the middle of writing this book) delivered eight puppies who brought us back to the early days of parenting where sleep deprivation ruled—the endless bowls of formula, kibble, and cleanup. Thanks for running the kids in all directions and staying up past your bedtime to let me complete "just one more recipe." You're my "Supper Man."

To my Girlie Pop, MacKenzie, you are the best distraction with your late evening visits, Taylor Swift songs on repeat, and storytelling practice that paid off when you brought home the title of Virginia's 2021 Forensics Storytelling State Champion during the writing of this book.

My "li'l man" William, I am so appreciative of the endless water and snacks to keep me fueled. You continuously make me laugh out loud when I need it, and I am so glad you have discovered the Beatles so you pop in to say, "What's poppin', Shorty?" and share their music on repeat. Way to go on scoring the highest Earth Sciences SOL in your school while I was writing recipes. I am proud of you!

Thank you, Abi, for the emails and photos that share your successes and remind me of the fire in my soul.

Louise, it has been a year! I have missed our daily phone calls and secret sharing. Thank you for still being my rock and loving me. I love you so very much.

To my Sister Squad, Kim and Tami: The texts that went all day and far into the night. The .gif wars on Facebook. And the impromptu trip you planned to visit me when my soul was on empty. I am so grateful the universe aligned for us to love each other. I love you BIG!!

Jake, thank you for your love and conversation. Sharing the story of your life, defeat, and success reminds me that even when it's hard, it's worth it. I am so thankful for your encouragement and our conversations.

Dad, I'm so glad I have you and your example. I love you.

To my mom and Charlotte the Great, for teaching me to cook.

Sherri, I adore you. You have made me laugh during this writing process and I love talking about (and eating) food with you! xoxo

A shout-out to everyone on the Callisto team who made this cookbook possible. Special thanks to Rebecca, who made me feel human when I was falling behind, and Caryn, my amazing editor who polished these recipes to perfection.

About the Author

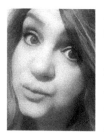 **Julee Morrison** is a blogger, wife, and mother of six who lives in the foothills of Virginia with their three dogs.

The *Complete College Cookbook* is her fourth cookbook. Her first book, *The Instant Pot® College Cookbook: 75 Quick and Easy Meals that Taste Like Home,* celebrates her family recipes and making quick meals everyone will love. *The How-To Cookbook for Teens* is a beginner cookbook with recipes to excite young chefs. *The Complete Cookbook for Teens: 120+ Recipes to Level Up Your Kitchen* teaches young adults a range of cooking skills through straightforward instructions, plenty of tips and tricks, and more than 120 easy recipes.

Her writing has appeared in HuffPost, Scary Mommy, PopSugar, SheKnows, Yahoo Shine, Love What Matters, and Ellen Nation, and her recipes have been featured in *Bon Appétit,* SparkPeople, and HuffPost.

Find Julee online at MommysMemorandum.com.